Energy Reset

Remove the Toxins
Reset Your Hormones
Restore Your Energy

Michelle L Brown, CTNC

© 2017 Michelle Brown.

All rights reserved. No part of this publication may be reproduced, distributed, or transmitted in any form or by any means, including photocopying, recording, or other electronic or mechanical methods, without the prior written permission of the publisher, except in the case of brief quotations embodied in reviews and certain other non-commercial uses permitted by copyright law.

Disclaimer: The information in this book is intended for reference purposes only and is not intended to diagnose, treat, or cure any disease. The information given here is designed to help you make informed decisions concerning your health and wellness. Consult your healthcare provider before undertaking any changes to your diet or health plan.

*This book is dedicated
to my children,
Shayla, Shelby and Dane.*

*You're the reason I do everything I do and
why
I want to show other moms
how important it is to
ditch the toxins and
regain their life.*

Bonus Materials

Don't forget to download the Bonuses to Energy Reset, including an exclusive interview with GMO experts, a coupon code for toxin-free skincare, the Energy Reset Diet Quick Start Guide and more!

Grab Your Bonuses Here:
www.overcomingauto.com/energyresetbonus

Table of Contents

Introduction

Is it just me, or does it seem like women today are struggling with their health like never before? In fact, I practically don't know a woman who isn't struggling on some level with nagging health issues that compromise her ability to be the person she wants to be and enjoy her life in a truly meaningful way.

From the mom with thyroid issues that leave her feeling exhausted, forgetful, and frumpy, to the grandmother whose rheumatoid arthritis is keeping her from enjoying even the simplest of tasks, it seems no one is immune to the health problems that rob women of their best years and leave them feeling constantly sick, exhausted, bloated, and fearful of the many diseases that are plaguing women today.

I wrote this book because I'm so *tired* of watching women struggle endlessly with the fatigue and frustration of hormonal imbalance and toxic overload—and, most of the time, they don't even know what is causing it.

Debilitating exhaustion, poor memory and concentration, depression, anxiety, digestive issues, thyroid problems, heavy periods that last for two weeks, cystic acne, dry skin, weight gain—you name it. Everywhere I look, I see women who are struggling with at least one, if not multiple, of these problems.

They share their woes with me over lunch at the park with the kids while munching on sugar-laden (but low-fat!) Greek yogurt—which they swear they could never give up because it's where they get "protein." They look so pretty, makeup in place, and perfume applied. All of which harbor secret toxins that are disrupting their delicate female hormones and even damaging DNA, which can lead to serious health issues like autoimmune disease. Yep, your beauty products really can do all that.

Unsuspectingly, they dutifully apply antibiotic-laden hand sanitizer to their children in an effort to keep nasty germs away that might make their little ones sick. Never mind the fact that hand sanitizer damages the gut microbiome and destroys the beneficial bacteria right along with the bad, leaving the immune system even more vulnerable to the onslaught of infectious agents she is trying to avoid in the first place.

I know women aren't doing these things because they don't care how it affects their health. In fact, I believe it's just the opposite. We're doing what we believe is best for ourselves and our families. Except that, in many cases, what we've been told is best is actually wrong. *Dead wrong.*

The thing is, most of the women I know are so amazing. They don't like to rock the boat and they want to believe the best in others and feel a sense of community with other women—all great qualities—which are also all expertly exploited by major corporations for their profit, *not yours.*

By now, you might be a little annoyed with me for disrespecting your lady-style. Look, I'm not some hippie, no makeup wearing, only-eat-organic-food-that-I-cooked-myself kinda girl. First of all, I love makeup. Thank God for makeup, because this momma needs all the help she can get, you know what I'm saying? And, while I definitely believe that organic is best, I'm also a real mom. I know how tough it can be to buy all organic, let alone cook from scratch. So, I'm not here to impose some "do or die" rules on you that just make life more stressful.

What I am against is all the lies the cosmetic industry tells unsuspecting women. This includes the lies the food industry, the pharmaceutical industry and, yes, even the government tells us in an effort to get us to buy their product, use their drugs (instead of truly healing our bodies) and to conform to public policy, which serves those major corporations more than it does the individual it should be protecting.

So, if you are going to be mad at someone, let's get mad at the companies that are unjustly selling us a package of lies right along with their toxic products. Besides, I'm going to share with you some amazing and easy alternatives to those toxic products that fill our bathroom and kitchen shelves. So, no worries. You'll still be looking beautiful and eating delicious meals that are quick and easy to prepare. You just won't be sacrificing your health and your hormones in the process.

Speaking of damaging your hormones, did you know that toxins are now thought to be the biggest driver of disease in the world today? Back in the day, Grandma didn't have to worry about endocrine disruptors from plastic bottles or heavy metal toxicity from eating contaminated tuna. She was more concerned with those infectious diseases that could strike without warning. My own great-grandmother's little sister died from an infection that started out as a simple blister on her foot. *Oh, how times have changed.*

While most of us don't have to worry about dying from an infected blister or contracting communicable diseases like typhoid fever, the truth is, we're much less healthy than great-grandma was. Assaulted by toxins on a daily basis, our immune systems are overworked and undernourished. Babies are born with an average of 200 chemicals in their umbilical cord blood—*at birth*. Toxins are already doing their dirty work within their precious, tiny bodies. And, if you've been on this planet longer than nine months, your toxic load is much higher.

We've got a problem, Mom. Yet, instead of sounding the alarm, raising the standard, and fighting against the odds, women are going along complacently, overloading their bodies with toxins, all because some company convinced them they should in the name of beauty, health, and of doing what any "good mom" would do.

I say it's time to take a stand, ladies. It's time to take a look at what we are really doing to our health and get to the root of the exhaustion, hormonal imbalance, and depression that way too many of us are up against and start taking back our birthright as healthy, strong, and truly beautiful women who can face life with faith and enthusiasm instead of fear and overwhelm.

As a mom who has struggled with my own health, I'm also concerned for my children's. Little did I know when I was a kid, the toxic foods I was eating, the dental work I had done, and my favorite Asian pear-scented body lotion I applied religiously in high school, were slowly, but, oh so surely, damaging my body in a way that I would come to pay for in a big way later in life. Now, I look at my three children and am determined to fight, not only for my own health and wholeness, but for theirs as well.

By the way, if you're not a mom, no worries. Everything I will be sharing with you in this book still applies whether you've had children or not. In fact, it applies whether you are even female or not. We're all suffering from a toxic burden that's slowly unraveling our health. Unfortunately, women tend to be more susceptible to the ravages of toxic overload than our male counterparts.

If you can relate to any of the health issues I've mentioned so far, then allow me to show you how toxins in our food, our environment, and even the toxic thoughts that keep us from feeling our best, are all contributing to your diminishing health, and how you can get back on track by taking down the toxins that are trying to take you out.

I really see what we're up against as women today as a fight for our lives Not only our lives, but our children's lives as well. Let me share with you how I went from a typical stay-at-home mom, silently suffering with thyroid disease, to a Certified Transformational Nutrition Coach with a mission to help women ditch the toxins that are robbing them of their best years so they can restore the hormonal balance that is so critical to healthy digestion, detoxification, and energy production.

Chapter 1
My Story

I know the frustration of living with overwhelming exhaustion.

I vividly remember standing in front of the bathroom mirror one morning, looking at my thinning hair and puffy face and knowing I felt exhausted, even though I had just woke up! I remember thinking, "I don't feel good. *I never feel good.*" It was truly a depressing moment.

I didn't know if I could ever feel better—and I was only in my early thirties. I had been diagnosed with hypothyroidism years earlier, early in my twenties, and had struggled with chronic health issues long before that. At one point, I asked my doctor why, since I was taking medication for an underactive thyroid, I still felt tired most of the time and still experienced a lot of hair loss. Her answer didn't give me much hope. "I think it's just never quite the same, even with the medication," she told me. In other words, "S*orry, sister. This is just the way things are.*"

I left the doctor's office that day feeling pretty hopeless. I didn't know there was a way to heal my body and be free from the ravages of chronic disease. I thought that I ate a healthy diet. I exercised. I didn't think I lived a particularly stressful life. And I knew, as a Christian, that God's plan for my life included a healthy mind and body. I just didn't know how to get it. There was so much I didn't know then that I know now. I *know* it's possible to regain your energy and lead a healthy and vibrant life. I know it's possible for me—and it's possible for you as well.

Let's Start at The Beginning

Like the typical child born in my generation, I was born via C-section and bottle-fed soy formula because I cried as an infant—All. The. Time. I grew up in an active family, but the standard American diet of fast food, junk food, and soda were, well, standard fare in my American home. All things that I would come to find out would impact my health much later in life.

When I reached my teen years, things really took a wrong turn. It was the early '90s and the low-fat craze was in full swing; a dietary fad that I, unfortunately, subscribed to with full on enthusiasm. To make matters worse, I suffered with eating disorders throughout my high school years; from anorexia, to bulimia, to binge eating. My relationship with food and with myself was at an all-time low and I wasn't even in my twenties yet.

My poor eating and lifestyle habits led to a full range of health issues: hair loss, horrible acne, amenorrhea, depression, digestive problems, pituitary issues, and more. I'm also convinced my thyroid problems began at this point, but I was never tested until years later. I was in my teens, but felt like I was an old woman.

In my twenties, things began to look up a bit. Though I never fully recovered from the symptoms of hair loss, fatigue, and acne, I began to take better care of myself. I finally had my thyroid hormone levels checked and began medication to make up for the thyroid hormones my body wasn't adequately producing. I recommitted my life to God my freshman year in college and, as a result, I experienced freedom from the eating disorders that had come to define my life. I began to take better care of myself. I began to eat better. I began to *feel* better.

Unfortunately, I adopted a mostly vegetarian diet that included processed soy foods like soy burgers and soy milk, as well as processed seed oils like canola oil. I thought these foods were better choices for me. Little did I know, they were contributing to my downward spiral into chronic autoimmune issues that wouldn't surface in full force until my early thirties.

Toxic foods weren't the only place where my immune system, slowly but surely, was being overwhelmed by toxins either. Little did I know, the drugstore skincare products I was using to keep my skin soft and clear were full of toxic chemicals that were contributing to my nosedive into hormonal self-destruction. Or, that making poor choices in my daily habits—like staying up late and stressing out about every little thing—were also pushing my weakened immune system further into a state of full on autoimmune disease.

After giving birth to my first child at the age of 25, I began to experience the frustrating and puzzling symptoms of thyroid disease that I didn't yet realize were the warning signs of some serious health issues. The months and years after childbirth are often a time when women begin to experience thyroid issues in full force and I was no exception. I began to have strange symptoms, including muscle pain in my arm and leg that never went away. When the pain moved to my thyroid area I began to suspect the root of my issues lay there and finally went to the doctor.

It was at that time I was told I had Hashimoto's thyroiditis. I was never told what that diagnosis meant. In fact, the doctor simply increased my dosage of thyroid hormone medication and that was that. In doing my own research, I learned that Hashimoto's is, in fact, an autoimmune disease where the immune system begins to attack the thyroid gland, eventually destroying it to the point that it cannot continue to make the thyroid hormones your body needs to function.

By the way, this is the typical way that autoimmune thyroid conditions are treated by conventional medical practitioners. You're simply given a prescription for a thyroid replacement hormone to make up for what your own thyroid gland can no longer produce and sent on your merry way without any explanation as to why your thyroid isn't functioning properly in the first place. But, let's not get ahead of ourselves here.

Fast forward a few years to the birth of my two youngest children when Hashimoto's finally reared its ugly head in full force. At the age of 32, a few months after my son was born, I began to experience a full on autoimmune attack: I began to lose weight rapidly (I barely weigh 100 lb soaking wet, so this was an alarming development for me.). My heart would begin to beat furiously, even when I was resting. I had constant diarrhea. The hair loss I had experienced from my teen years reached a fever pitch. I could run my hand through my hair and pull out a handful of hair at a time.

Oh, and I haven't even mentioned the cognitive issues that plagued me throughout my years of poor health: general fatigue and "brain fog" that many women experience, to more alarming issues, like the inability to control my thoughts and the unexplained irritability and frustration that I did my best to hide behind my quiet, low-key nature. It was time to see the doctor again.

While my symptoms were extremely alarming to me, my doctor seemed unconcerned. A quick lab test confirmed that Hashimoto's was in full swing, but my doctor didn't particularly feel the need to do anything about it. I finally asked if she would at least change my thyroid hormone medication to a different brand in hopes that it might relieve my symptoms. She finally agreed, and I was switched from Synthroid to Armour Thyroid, which did, indeed, put a stop to all of the strange symptoms I had begun to experience.

I was frustrated, and a little hurt, that my doctor seemed so unconcerned by my symptoms. I want to make it clear at this point, that I have nothing against doctors or the medical establishment, in particular. However, I did learn a lesson from this, and, I hope, if you take anything away from my story, it is that you must be your own advocate for your health care. Do your own research and, while I would never tell you to ignore the advice of your doctor, I believe you should follow your instincts and make the decision that is right for you.

After changing my medication, I wish I could say that my struggles with autoimmune disease ended there, but they didn't. Anyone who understands autoimmune issues can understand why. Whether an autoimmune disease manifests itself as thyroid disease, Crohn's disease, fibromyalgia, multiple sclerosis, or any of hundreds of manifestations of autoimmunity, the root cause is all the same: an immune system gone haywire so that it begins to attack the very body it is meant to protect.

The conventional treatment for most autoimmune issues involves treating the disease with drugs that suppress the immune system to the point that it no longer attacks the body. Or, in the case of thyroid autoimmune disease, to simply replace the hormones the body is no longer able to make in hope that the individual can function as normally as possible.

As one researcher on the forefront of thyroid autoimmune disease, Dr. Izabella Wentz, puts it, this is like trying to fill a leaking cup. Adding thyroid hormone via medication may help to alleviate the symptoms, but it does nothing to fix the root of the problem. This is why most people with autoimmune issues continue to steadily grow worse over time. But, I'm getting ahead of myself again.

After switching to Armour Thyroid medication, I felt somewhat better. But, I never felt really great. I was always tired, but I thought that was just normal for me. I just wasn't one of those high energy people that could get a lot done. I needed a nap almost every day just to function. I'd learned to accept thyroid disease, and the low energy and brain fog that came with it, as my new normal. Until one fateful day.

The Turning Point

I can tell you exactly when the turning point came for me. I was surfing the internet, scouring one of my favorite sites for healthy recipes. I've always been a bit of a health nut and love to cook. That day, as I pulled up my favorite website on clean eating, I was amazed to read an article published by the author on her recent thyroid disease diagnosis.

She didn't know a lot about the condition at that point, being newly diagnosed, but she had already learned three things that I had never learned in more than a decade of living with thyroid health issues. She had learned to avoid three things in her diet that were contributing to thyroid dysfunction: gluten, dairy products, and soy.

I was blown away. What?! Gluten, dairy products, and soy could be the cause of all my years of misery? The article linked to several websites on treating thyroid disease naturally, which I devoured, reading everything I could on how food affected my thyroid health, as well as things like toxins and a lack of sleep. From these sites, I learned that thyroid disease could indeed be overcome, even reversed, in some cases, and that some of the very foods I thought were good for me were anything but. (Whole grains! Bad for you? Who knew?).

I sat at my computer in a state of shock that day. Honestly, I don't even remember most of what those websites said. But, I do know that, for the first time in years, I felt hope. I knew things could be different.

I'd like to say that I immediately removed gluten, dairy, and soy from my diet and that everything changed instantly. That wasn't the case. While changing my diet was a major step forward, my road to freedom was paved with ups and downs. It took time to heal my gut and deal with underlying infections that were inciting inflammation in my body and ramping up the autoimmune response. I started replacing toxic, chemical-laden beauty products with natural alternatives that didn't derail my hormones. I had to learn to relax and rest so my body could heal. Something that didn't come easily for my Type A personality.

I finally learned that *food could be extremely powerful in healing the body* and that ditching the toxins in my home would reduce the toxic load that was irritating my weakened immune system. That certain habits, like getting enough sleep, exercise, and sunshine—seemingly simple things—could have a powerful effect on my body's healing response. I learned to take better care of myself, eat the right foods, and nourish not only my body, but my soul as well. I also became a Certified Transformational Nutrition Coach (CTNC) so that I could help other women who are feeling stuck in the same place I was to radically transform their health and regain their energy.

I would like to invite you to travel this road with me. In *Energy Reset,* I will be your guide to unraveling the root cause of those annoying health issues that are plaguing women everywhere today: from the road signs that point to the issues at the root of your fatigue, to the pit stops along the way that are keeping you from feeling your best. My hope is that you will learn through my own experience, not only how to take better care of your body and step into the health you desire, but also how to take responsibility for your choices so you can experience the life you were meant to live.

After all, health in and of itself isn't the only reason you want to embark on this journey. I know you want to regain your health and energy so that you can show up in your own life the way you know you were meant to. So you can be the wonderful woman, amazing wife, and great friend you want to be. So you can lose the frustration that you can't be the great mom you were meant to be because you are just too exhausted and irritable to be there for your kids like you want to.

Or, to overcome the fear that you might not be there to watch your kids grow up and experience life with you cheering them on.

Maybe you secretly feel ashamed that you're not the wife that your spouse needs you to be because exhaustion, depression, or anxiety are keeping you locked inside yourself.

Whatever your reason for starting this journey, I want you to feel today that you hold in your hands the key that will release you from the prison of exhaustion, brain fog, and hormonal imbalance so you can take the journey toward health and wholeness in every area. As a certified health coach, I will be here to cheer you along on your journey, pointing out the pitfalls ahead, and helping you make a game plan to get your life back on track. Are you ready? Let's do this!

Chapter 2
Why So Tired?

Fatigued. Tired. Run down. Exhausted. Do any of these words sound familiar? Far too many women live these words on a daily basis, frustrated that they feel so exhausted, yet unsure what to do about it. If you picked up this book, chances are, you're one of them.

Maybe you believe, like I did for years, you just aren't a "high-energy person." Many women are told by their otherwise loving family and friends, who don't understand the depth of fatigue she's experiencing, that she's just lazy—or worse—*crazy*.

Perhaps you've been told that, or maybe even believed it about yourself. You know life has more to offer and that you're capable of so much more—but you are just too tired to go after it.

Fatigue can run the gamut from feeling a little sleepy after lunch to full-blown exhaustion that leaves you weak and helpless after completing even the simplest tasks. If you've ever had to lay down on the couch for an hour because taking laundry out of the dryer just about did you in, you know the deep-seated exhaustion I'm talking about.

For others, fatigue can be a relatively minor, yet equally frustrating, condition to be battled on a daily basis. Countless men and women can relate to the afternoon slump, to waking up tired after a full night's sleep, or that oh—so-maddening condition known as "brain fog" that can leave you feeling irritable, confused, and unable to think clearly, as if you're trying to think through a fog (hence the term, *brain fog*).

When fatigue becomes a daily occurrence that lasts for years, we often stop wondering what's wrong, assuming this is just the way we are and no longer questioning whether or not fatigue will be a part of your day—because it just is. Yet, deep down, you know that this constant companion called exhaustion is an unwanted guest who's overstayed its welcome.

Yet, how do you give fatigue the eviction notice? You want your life back, but fatigue is like a wicked stepmother who seems to hold the upper hand. You want your life back—*your body back*—but you're simply not sure what it takes to get there.

Thankfully, you can get "there"—to a place where you have plenty of energy to function on a daily basis while enjoying your life and thinking clearly. Before you can get there, however, you've got to ditch the fatigue and what's causing it, so your body can function optimally again.

Fatigue is always a sign of a greater underlying issue. The root of that underlying issue can take some detective work to unravel, however. It will likely require changes to your diet and lifestyle that may not be easy at first. Yet, they're *so* worth it. The things you give up in order to gain your sanity, your energy, and your life are nothing in comparison to the reward.

What exactly is daily exhaustion robbing you of, by the way? Have you ever really stopped to take stock of just what living in a fog of fatigue and confusion is costing you?

The Nefarious Effects of Fatigue

Difficulty Concentrating

Ever had an important report due at work but you just can't seem to wrap your head around it and get it pulled off on time? Or, maybe it was your turn to bring treats to your kiddo's weekly playgroup and you dropped the ball—*again.*

Can't remember where you placed your keys or what you changed your email password to just yesterday? Difficulty concentrating is par for the course when you're exhausted. While we all have a few moments, here and there, where our memory lapses, it can be alarming when it becomes the norm rather than the exception.

Some forgetfulness can be relatively harmless, while other times it can have disastrous consequences. I don't think I'll ever forget the article I read in *Parents* magazine several years ago about a woman whose young child died when she accidentally left him in the car while she was at work one especially hot day. I know what you're thinking—*Who forgets their child in the backseat of a hot car for hours?* An exhausted mom who's too tired to think straight, that's who. After a sleepless night caring for a sick older sibling this otherwise loving mother was too exhausted to remember to drop off her toddler at daycare on the way to work. By the time she realized what she had done, it was too late.

Most of the time, our tendency towards forgetfulness doesn't have life or death consequences. But, it can mean the slow death of our career when we can't concentrate on important tasks in the workplace. Friendships can be damaged when we trade our loving concern for our friends for mind-numbing fatigue.

Brain fog is a relatively new term coined to define the condition of the human mind that many men and women are suffering from these days. While brain fog can sound like a somewhat vague notion, if you can relate to feeling like you're "in a fog" and can't seem to keep your focus—welcome to brain fog.

Difficulty Completing Tasks

You know the laundry needs done, the dog needs a bath, and your family is asking,

"What's for dinner?" but, you're *just.so.tired.* Fatigue can often leave women feeling like they don't have the mental or physical energy left to complete even the basic tasks of life.

If you're a mom like me, you can probably relate to the never ending to-do list that only seems to grow longer with each passing day. You do your best to check items off your to do list, but life just seems so overwhelming sometimes. The results of not being able to keep up with the daily demands of life can lead to a downward spiral of emotions—from overwhelm to hopelessness to depression.

I've personally been the mom who struggled to stay on my feet after even the simplest tasks, like making my kids breakfast or folding laundry. My to-do list didn't dwindle simply because I was too tired to keep up either. In fact, it just grew longer as my time was spent lying on the couch, trying to recover just enough to take care of the basic needs of my young children. Life doesn't wait just because you are tired.

A good support network of family and friends who are willing and able to help you pick up the slack can make a world of difference.

However, for most women the burden of housework, paying bills, cooking, and taking care of children falls squarely on their shoulders. Because we think we should be supermom, we find it difficult to ask for help when we need to. The negative emotions of overwhelm and frustration only add to the stress that negatively impacts our health. Thus begins the downward spiral.

Difficulty in Relationships

When my kids were toddlers (and, truth be told, sometimes even now), missing a nap was a recipe for a major meltdown. Too tired and cranky to control their emotions any longer, they would wail with frustration at the slightest provocation, sometimes lashing out angrily when they didn't get their way. Normally sweet-tempered and lovable, they could turn into little monsters when they were overtired, stressing out everyone around them in the process.

It's a problem that is easy to identify in little ones. You've probably seen a loving momma making excuses for her temper-tantrum-throwing toddler at the grocery store or church. "He needs his nap," she might excuse, as she drags a sleepy toddler from the room kicking and screaming. While we can understand how kiddos lose it when they haven't had enough rest, it's not nearly as cute or as easy to excuse when it comes to the grown-up set.

Unfortunately, we don't necessarily outgrow our tendency towards crankiness when we feel exhausted. And those around us might not be as willing to understand—or excuse—our theatrics when we give into the urge to let our emotions rule our responses. The unfortunate consequence of all this fatigue-induced irritability can often be negatively felt in our relationships with those closest to us.

Hopefully, you aren't still kicking and screaming on the floor when you don't get your way like you might have done when you were two. But, stop and think of how the fatigue you cope with day after day often goes hand in hand with a low emotional threshold, resulting in a range of emotions from sadness to anger and frustration. The inability to regulate our emotions has a serious impact on our relationships. Constantly grumping at friends and family will likely result in a desire to avoid you.

Even if your emotions aren't ruling you, your fatigue can impact your relationships in other ways. Many women have missed out on important milestones in their loved ones' lives due to debilitating fatigue that has left them unable to participate in even the most basic daily tasks—from reading a bedtime story to their children, to missing out on Grandma's 85th birthday party. And we haven't even talked about your sex life yet! Fatigue has far too many women living with less than fulfilling relationships.

Difficulty Controlling Emotions

Speaking of temper tantrums, the end result of all this fatigue can be emotions that only perpetuate the cycle of exhaustion. We feel too tired to keep up with the demands of life, so we feel overwhelmed. Feelings of overwhelm often result in losing sight of the bigger picture and difficulty seeing workable solutions to the problem at hand. Overwhelm spirals into feelings of guilt, frustration, disappointment, and, eventually, anger, resentment, and depression. These emotions only serve to deplete our energy stores and we fall even further behind, struggle even more with taking action, and even misplace the hope that keeps us moving forward in tough times.

Whew! Who knew exhaustion could be so costly? I'm guessing you do, if it's something you've lived with for any length of time. Fortunately, there is a way out of the cycle of fatigue—overwhelm—frustration—depression that so many women are up against these days.

Let me emphatically state that again: Exhaustion is NOT supposed to be your normal way of life. You were created to be energetic, emotionally balanced, mentally alert, and filled with peace. I lived with debilitating fatigue for so long that, to be honest, I lost sight of God's plan for my life and felt afraid that this state of weakness and overwhelm was just going to be my new normal. Fortunately, I learned otherwise. If that is where you're at, I can promise you it's not supposed to be your normal either. You can give fatigue the boot, feel amazing, and regain your health and energy.

What's *Really* at the Root of Fatigue?

What does it really take to ditch the fatigue and brain fog anyways? Because exhaustion is a symptom of an underlying issue with your health, it's important to look for what's *really* driving the cycle of never-ending fatigue, and not just try to mask the symptoms with quick fixes (Yes, I'm talking about you, coffee.)

Whether fatigue is a minor annoyance or a major crisis for you, the root cause is the same as it is for all manner of disease and ill health we may experience and I like to sum it up in one word—**toxins.** Toxins are those things in our diet and lifestyle that harm the body and mind, causing damage to cells and wreaking havoc on our ability to cope with life successfully.

While the scientific definition of a toxin is a little more precise, many healthcare professionals have come to use the term to refer to *anything* that can harm us—from toxins in our food and skincare products, to toxic thoughts that keep us stuck in our efforts to move forward in life. Yep, toxins can invade every part of your life. Your level of fatigue is simply a clue to just how overloaded your body has become with the toxins that flood our lives today.

In the following chapters, we'll dive into five areas where toxins are keeping you sluggish and overwhelmed and find solutions that leave you feeling your best: energetic, clear-minded, and emotionally stable. We'll ditch the toxins in the following five areas so you can finally start to feel alive again and experience vibrant health:

Toxic Foods – No matter how well you eat, chances are that you have some foods in your diet that are devoid of the nutrients we need to feel our best. Not only that, some foods directly contribute to leaky gut (which we'll look at in just a moment) and increase inflammation within the body. It simply isn't possible to overestimate the power of food to heal and nourish your body and even affect your mental health. I'll show you exactly which foods to eat—and which to avoid—to ditch the exhaustion fast.

Toxic Chemicals – Are some of your favorite health and beauty products disrupting your hormones and leaving you feeling exhausted and miserable? Despite the cosmetic industry's pie-in-the-sky promise of "visibly younger looking skin", many of the chemicals in these miracle concoctions are known endocrine disruptors and carcinogens. *True story*. Same goes for many cleaning products and other synthetic chemicals that have been marketed to you in the name of a cleaner, fresher home. No worries, though. I'm not asking you to ditch makeup altogether. Thankfully, there are some amazing products on the market that actually deliver on their promises of healthier, younger looking skin—toxin free! Likewise, you can clean your home just as effectively without the use of toxic chemicals and keep your hormones happy while you're at it.

Toxic Thoughts – Your thoughts matter. Research into how thoughts affect our health have actually shown that our thoughts can change our DNA. We'll look at which types of thoughts are defeating you mentally and physically, and how to choose the best thoughts that will have you feeling strong and powerful in no time. (Hint—It all starts with God's Word!)

Toxic Habits – Some of the simple things we do every day without even thinking about it can contribute to fatigue and overwhelm. No matter how well you have dialed in your nutrition or detoxed your home of chemicals, if you don't have these habits firmly in place, you could very likely be stalling your progress towards vibrant energy and, even, weight loss. We will learn to identify bad habits and easily change them in three key areas that will turn you into an energy powerhouse.

Toxic Infections – Many women today are dealing with underlying infections due to the unhealthy state of the standard American diet and poor gut health. When your energy levels don't respond to changes in the way you eat, think, and live, it's time to consider if an unknown infection is at work. We'll look at the clues to whether or not a chronic gut infection is undermining your health and what to do if you suspect that might be the case for you.

Whether the fatigue you are dealing with is mild or severe, the good news is—yes, I'll say it again—it can change. No matter how difficult fatigue is to deal with, ditching the toxins in these five areas will help you to quickly regain your energy and rest your hormones. Before we dive into ditching the toxins in these areas, however, let's look at exactly how toxins drain our energy and, not only leave us feeling exhausted, but contribute to major health issues, including autoimmune diseases and cancer. Here's a clue: **It all begins in the gut.**

How Do Toxins Do Their Dirty Work?

From movies like, *Honey, I Shrunk the Kids,* to the story of *Thumbelina,* we humans love to imagine what it would be like to see the world from a bug's eye view. It can be hard to relate to the microscopic world, let alone the insect world, since we can't, well, *see it.* In fact, before the invention of the microscope, and before things like bacteria and microscopic amoeba were discovered, humans scoffed at the idea that tiny, microscopic life forms were responsible for ill health. With an unfortunate lack of knowledge of how viruses and bacteria caused disease, doctors even discredited the idea of washing their hands before treating patients, despite the fact that evidence showed it dramatically cut down on the number of patient deaths.

Ever heard the story? In 1846, Dr. Ignaz Semmelweis, a doctor at the maternity ward of the Vienna General Hospital, noticed something interesting. While the women whose births were attended by midwives usually fared well after their deliveries, those who were attended by physicians often had a very different outcome. In fact, the women who were attended by the physicians had a much greater chance of dying from puerperal fever (also known as childbed fever)—five times greater, as a matter of fact.

A man ahead of his time, Dr. Semmelweis wanted to find out what caused such a high rate of deaths in these women. After much observation, trial, and error, Dr. Semmelweis discovered that the physicians often attended the childbirth after coming straight from working on cadavers of women who had died from puerperal fever—without washing their hands. *Yeah, I know.*

It's obvious to us now that the physicians were transporting the very infectious bacteria that had killed the cadavers straight back to the laboring women. But, back in those days, the concept of washing one's hands to eradicate infections was considered somewhat radical. Which is just what Dr. Semmelweis proposed—even going so far as *proving* that properly sterilizing the instruments used for childbirth and hand washing dramatically reduced the number of deaths from puerperal fever. Unfortunately, the other physicians summarily dismissed Dr. Semmelweis' recommendations and continued to attend to childbirth without proper sanitation. Scores of women suffered and died as a result.

While this story seems absurd to us now, given what we know about germs, I think it illustrates an important lesson about human nature that we would do well to take note of. **What we can't see or don't understand, we tend to discredit**. I bring this up because I think it's one of the reasons so many are struggling with their health today. Sure, we know that toxins are bad for us. That cleaning with toxic chemicals is probably damaging to our health. That the mercury fillings in our mouth aren't exactly good for us. Yet, we continue to ignore those facts, and the annoying signs of disease they are creating in our body. Many times, until it's too late.

If you could see what those toxins were doing to your body on the cellular level, however, you'd be singing a different tune. Remember that old '80s flick, *Inner Space*, where Dennis Quaid's character gets shrunken down and injected into the body of a store clerk played by Martin Short? (See, told you we love the idea of shrinking!) Let's pretend for a moment that we get to ride along with Dennis in his mini submarine, only this time, we're interested in locating the toxins circulating in our system and finding out exactly how they are damaging our cells.

Leaky Gut

Let's say, as we're cruising through the human body, we end up in the digestive tract where food is digested and broken down in order to assimilate the nutrients we need to grow and repair tissues. Amongst all the tiny particles of peas, carrots, and beef from the stew you had for lunch are also particles of the cornbread you ate. As these particles are broken down into individual molecules of proteins, fats, and carbohydrates, they attach to specialized cells located on the lining of the intestine wall so that your body can assimilate the nutrients into energy for your body.

These specialized gut cells, called *enterocytes*, are responsible for keeping out foreign invaders—toxins and pathogens that we ingest when we eat—as well as letting in the nutrients from the foods we eat. When things are working properly, it's a beautiful system that keeps us healthy and thriving. When things go awry, toxins get a free pass to enter the bloodstream and wreak havoc on the cells of your body, from the brain to the big toe. We call this unfortunate situation "leaky gut" and, due to our constant assault of toxins in modern life, it's alarmingly common.

Interestingly, this lining of our gut wall is only one cell thick. That's not much of a barrier between us and the outside world. While certain things, like nutrients, were meant to get through, certain factors can cause the cells of the gut wall to become more permeable than they should. This is why leaky gut is more technically referred to as "increased intestinal permeability".

When the enterocytes become damaged through exposure to toxins that harm the gut (Such as the gluten protein in that cornbread you just ate), the gut lining can form holes that allow the contents of the gut to leak into the bloodstream—and into the arms of the resident immune cells that are awaiting any foreign invaders on the other side of the gut wall.

The space in-between the enterocytes is where leaky gut happens as well. Normally, these cells line up tightly next to one another, like soldiers standing guard. This space in-between the enterocytes—called *tight junctions*—keeps anything from crossing the intestinal lining. However, certain things can trigger the tight junctions to lose their integrity and, suddenly, everything gets a free pass into your bloodstream—including toxins.

So, let's think this through: When the gut lining, which normally absorbs nutrients while keeping everything else out, becomes damaged and full of holes (leaky), you've suddenly got everything and anything that was and wasn't supposed to crossing the gut barrier where immune cells are waiting to protect your body from any threats. This constant barrage of toxins keeps the immune system on high alert 24/7 and leads to chronic inflammation, which, as we'll see in the next chapter, has a domino effect on nearly every other function and system of the body, including hormonal health. This, my friend, is a bird's eye view (or rather, a microscopic view) of how toxins are keeping you sick, exhausted, and depressed. *You're welcome.*

The Gut Microbiome

We can't talk about the gut without mentioning the *gut microbiome*. These are the trillions of microbes that live in your digestive tract. These tiny microorganisms that live in the gut—as well as on the skin, in the mouth and other surfaces of the body—have a very special relationship with us, their human host, that includes boosting immunity, synthesizing certain key nutrients, and even breaking down dangerous toxins such as heavy metals and pesticides, as we'll see later.

The microbiome is composed of a very diverse mini universe of bacteria, yeasts, and viruses, and each person's gut microbiome is as uniquely different as their fingerprints. This includes beneficial, as well as pathogenic, organisms and the end goal is to have a diverse gut flora of beneficial bacteria that keeps the bad guys in check. When something goes awry, however, the "bad guys" are quick to take over. Like a hostage situation gone wrong, they bully the beneficial bacteria, crowding them out and taking over territory, while releasing toxic waste products into the environment—your gut.

Guess what the good guys—your beneficial bacteria—like to have around in order to thrive? Fiber, healthy fats, and proteins from nutrient dense foods, plenty of clean pure air, and water. Guess what the bad guys thrive on? You guessed it, plenty of toxic foods like sugar, grains, and dairy. Toxins damage the delicate balance of microbes in the gut, which weakens the immune system and leaves us depleted of certain key nutrients that are necessary for energy production.

Ever taken an antibiotic only to end up with a nasty case of diarrhea? If so, you've experienced first-hand how vital a healthy gut microbiome is to good digestion. Because antibiotics are equal opportunity destroyers, they kill off the beneficial bacteria right along with the pathogens they're supposed to be eradicating. Your doctor might have recommended a probiotic, or eating some yogurt to help offset the effects of the antibiotics. Unfortunately, many of the beneficial bacteria in the gut simply don't bounce back after a round of antibiotics, especially when coupled with the fact that the standard American diet and the constant influx of toxins further damage the gut flora.

That's a rather unfortunate situation since a healthy gut microbiome may well be the most important factor in staying healthy and keeping inflammation and toxic overload to a minimum. Not only do these bacteria synthesize B vitamins, vitamin K, facilitate the absorption of dietary fatty acids, and aid in the absorption of key minerals, they also play an important role in properly developing and regulating the immune system and even influence genetic expression by switching genes off and on.

We'll take a closer look at the gut microbiome and how to keep it healthy in coming chapters, but I want to mention it here so that you'll start thinking of your gut microbiome—and how the choices you make in what you put in and on your body are affecting this very vital part of your health.

When Toxins Move Beyond the Gut

Surprised to learn just how vital gut health is to living a fit, energetic life? If you're like I was, you probably never gave a second thought to how what was going on in your gut was playing out in your energy levels. Or, how the toxic foods you were eating were taxing the liver and disrupting your hormones. Who knew your gut was home to trillions of microbes that were directly responsible for keeping your immune system strong? Now that we know how toxins damage the gut lining and put the immune system on hyperalert, let's look at what happens as toxins move beyond the gut wall and into the bloodstream where they are carried to other parts of the body, including the thyroid, brain, and liver.

In the next chapter, we'll see how, once toxins breach the gut lining and make it to the immune tissue waiting on the other side, the battle really begins. The immune cells combat the toxins that are infiltrating the gut in an attempt to neutralize them. Unfortunately, in our toxic world, this never-ending job can be totally overwhelming for the immune system and that's when toxins can start making their way into the bloodstream—and, from there, every other part of your body.

This constant cycle of toxicity and inflammation is what leads to chronic health issues, including autoimmune diseases as your poor, overworked immune system, in a desperate attempt to eliminate the foreign invaders, begins to attack everything in sight, including your own body tissues. This all plays out in a complex system regulated by your hormones which we'll dive into in the next chapter. Many women dealing with exhaustion and hormonal issues may be wondering if they have a sluggish thyroid, or, perhaps, it's adrenal fatigue they've heard about. In the next chapter, we'll see exactly what happens as toxins move beyond the gut and begin to interfere with other systems of the body, including the thyroid, adrenals, and the brain.

Chapter 3
Beyond the Gut

Hormonal Woes in the Thyroid, Adrenals, Brain, and Immune System

So, now we know what's at the root of your debilitating fatigue, weight gain, brain fog, and moodiness—*toxins*. And, we know that those toxins disrupt your delicate hormonal balance and inflame the immune system by damaging the gut. Still, how does this translate into *your* fatigue? Maybe you've been asking yourself, "Is it a thyroid disorder? Adrenal fatigue? Fibromyalgia or chronic fatigue syndrome? Toxic mom-itis?" (Just kidding.) Knowing that toxins are damaging your immune system is one thing. Let's take a look at how the accumulation of toxins within the body affects those systems that directly translate into your level of energy, your mood, your ability to lose weight, and even your ability to think clearly.

Your Thyroid and Toxins

We can't talk about energy balance in the body without bringing up the little butterfly-shaped gland that resides at the base of the neck—your thyroid. Thyroid disease has reached epidemic proportions in the U.S today, and women are far more susceptible than men to struggle with the debilitating fatigue and mood issues that having a thyroid disorder practically guarantees. While it can be frustrating and disheartening to struggle with thyroid issues (or worse, have all the symptoms and, yet, be told that your thyroid hormone levels are "normal"), I think it's important to recognize that the thyroid gland is a highly sensitive organ and is one of the first places you're likely to see signs of distress within the body. And, that's a good thing. Here's why:

While debilitating fatigue can feel overwhelming, think of it simply as your body's way of telling you to slow down, focus on your health, and rest. It's almost as if the thyroid was meant to be an alarm system in the body, warning us when the toxic load has become too much and signaling us to take a closer look at our health. Dealing with thyroid disease certainly isn't fun. But, I want to encourage you to be thankful for your thyroid. Be thankful that your thyroid is sending you signals that things are out of balance so that you can make the corrections you need to make now before an even more serious issue presents itself down the road. Which, by the way, is very likely if you continue to ignore the warning signs your thyroid, your gut, and your immune system are trying to send you.

If you're already aware that your thyroid isn't functioning optimally, you may be surprised to learn that conventional medicine tends to get it all wrong when it comes to managing thyroid disorders. Whether you're struggling with hypothyroidism (an underactive thyroid), hyperthyroidism (an overactive thyroid), Hashimoto's thyroiditis, or Grave's disease (both autoimmune conditions that affect the thyroid), the truth is, almost all thyroid issues women deal with today *are* autoimmune in nature. Why is the thyroid so susceptible to attack from your own immune system?

The thyroid is responsible, with help from the pituitary gland and hypothalamus in the brain, for producing hormones which carefully regulate energy production in the body. Every cell in your body has receptors for thyroid hormones. This is why, when your thyroid is under producing, you can feel sluggish, cold, and experience constipation (slow digestion), and weight gain. Your thyroid simply isn't able to keep up with the constant demand for energy each and every cell requires to function optimally.

When your immune system is under assault from toxins on a continual basis, the thyroid is often one of the first organs to come under attack. Certain toxins, such as gluten, have been shown to closely resemble thyroid tissue. We'll look at gluten more closely in another chapter, but suffice it to say for now that, when this toxic protein enters the bloodstream by way of a leaky gut, your immune system goes on the attack, desperately trying to eradicate the threat of gluten and anything that closely resembles it.

This is where your thyroid gland gets caught in the crossfire and slowly, over time, the damage leads to a loss in production of that oh-so-important thyroid hormone. Because this process happens over time, this explains why you can begin to feel the effects of thyroid damage long before your doctor can find anything wrong with your thyroid hormone levels. That's assuming doc is even running the right tests, which is often not the case. But, that's a story for another day.

Gluten isn't the only toxin that damages the thyroid either. Fluoride, a chemical added to nearly every municipal drinking water system in the U.S., competes with iodine for uptake by the thyroid. While iodine is essential in the production of thyroid hormones, fluoride is a bit of a bully molecule, crowding out iodine and taking its place within the thyroid and effectively guaranteeing that you won't be able to produce adequate amounts of thyroid hormones.

To make matters even more complicated, the production of thyroid hormones requires adequate amounts of other important nutrients besides iodine—selenium and vitamin C, to name just a few. When we are depleted of these critical nutrients, because our damaged digestive systems can't properly absorb the nutrients from our food (that's if we are even consuming adequate nutrients in our diet, which usually doesn't happen), the thyroid takes another hit. Without the proper nutrients needed to produce thyroid hormones, it's really no wonder women in our nutrient depleted society are struggling with thyroid health by the millions.

By the way, these are just a *few* examples of how the thyroid gland is assaulted on a daily basis by the deluge of toxins in our modern world. There are many other toxins besides gluten and fluoride that have been shown to interfere with thyroid function, such as heavy metals and infectious bacteria. Your thyroid is one overworked and underappreciated little gland.

The Adrenals Get Involved

Your thyroid isn't the only organ that takes a hit under a constant barrage of toxins. All that inflammation put out by your immune system doesn't go unnoticed by the rest of the body. As you might imagine, when you are constantly under attack from toxins in your diet and environment, it puts a huge amount of stress on the body. When you are in a state of chronic stress, another oh-so-delicate hormonal pathway can go awry as well. Enter HPA-Axis dysregulation or what most people just call *adrenal fatigue.*

The "HPA" in HPA-Axis stand for the hypothalamus, pituitary, and adrenals and, just like with the thyroid, the hypothalamus and pituitary are command central in the brain for regulating the amount of hormones produced by the adrenal glands in response to environmental stimuli. Only in this case, instead of thyroid hormones, we're talking about cortisol—your resident stress hormone.

When your immune system is constantly bombarded by the stress of toxins, the hypothalamus gets the message to produce more cortisol! Quick! Bad things are happening and you need to stress out! Which might be a good thing if you're being chased by a rabid dog, for example. But, when that signal just keeps coming and coming to continually produce cortisol, sooner or later your poor little adrenals can't keep up and, suddenly, your body either can't make enough cortisol to even function normally *or* it's producing the right amount of hormone—just at the wrong time.

That's when women begin to experience the full-blown effects of adrenal fatigue, which include: exhaustion (obviously), weight gain (especially around the abdomen), anxiety and/or depression, irritability, brain fog, difficulty falling asleep or staying asleep at night, sugar cravings, or frequent thirst. All these signs point to unhappy adrenal glands that are overtaxed from an overload of toxins and stress and a lack of essential nutrients.

In his book, *The Adrenal Reset Diet*, Dr. Alan Christianson explains how adrenal fatigue can run the gamut from *stressed* to *wired and tired* where you may feel fatigue, yet be unable to fully relax, to the full-on exhaustion and weakness associated with the *crashed* level of adrenal fatigue where your body's ability to keep up with the constant demands of stress have depleted the adrenals to the point of no longer being able to adequately produce cortisol. If you're the person who needs a daily nap just to function normally, or ten hours of sleep a night doesn't even begin to alleviate the fatigue you battle constantly—welcome to the world of crashed adrenals.

The Adrenals—Not Just for Stress

The adrenals do more than just pump out cortisol, by the way. The sex hormones are also produced in the adrenal glands as well:

progesterone, testosterone, and estrogen. For many women who are struggling with adrenal dysfunction, estrogen dominance can further complicate matters. Estrogen dominance can pose many of the same symptoms of adrenal fatigue, such as difficulty losing weight, fatigue, anxiety, and moodiness. Got a spare tire around your middle that won't budge no matter what you do? You can thank excess estrogen for that.

Of course, estrogen is an important and essential hormone, especially for us ladies. So, what's the big deal about a little extra estrogen (besides having a little extra weight)? Left unchecked, excess estrogen can lead to some serious problems, including increased risk for diabetes, depression, and cancer. In a healthy woman, estrogen levels are kept in check by another sex hormone known as progesterone. Interestingly, progesterone is a precursor to cortisol.

When your body's need for cortisol goes up, so does your need for progesterone, leaving you depleted of this important hormone. When progesterone production is dampened, not only will you experience estrogen dominance, but your body will produce insufficient cortisol as well and will, once again, struggle to keep up with the constant demand for more progesterone. It's a vicious cycle and I'm betting you're beginning to see why getting off the toxin overload roller coaster will do amazing things for your health and energy levels.

As if your poor, overworked adrenals didn't have enough to do, they also have the responsibility of regulating blood sugar along with a little help from their old friend, the pancreas. As we've already seen, no aspect of your health and hormones exists in a vacuum. You simply can't be experiencing the destructive effects of adrenal fatigue without your blood sugar levels paying a price as well.

As we've already learned, cortisol is released in response to stress—whether it be psychological or physical—and cortisol, in turn, "talks" to the pancreas, suppressing the release of insulin, the hormone responsible for regulating blood sugar levels, in response to stress.

Insulin is a critical hormone in the regulation of body fat storage and energy levels. Many women struggling with adrenal issues and the blood sugar regulation issues that go along with it, have difficulty losing weight (no matter how hard they try), experience irritability when meals are missed, and other mood issues. I'm sure the term "hangry" was coined to describe a hormone depleted mom whose tanked blood sugar levels made her a bit, shall we say, grumpy. Ask me how I know. Left unchecked, blood sugar problems can develop into diabetes, heart disease, and cancer. This is one hormone you don't want to mess with, lady.

This is Your Brain on Toxins

While being constantly exhausted and feeling run down can be frustrating, the changes to mood and memory that inevitably accompany toxicity can be downright alarming. From moodiness, irritability, and forgetfulness to depression and anxiety, when you're "not yourself" it can be a scary feeling.

If sales of antidepressants are any indication, women are suffering with psychiatric dysfunction at nearly epidemic levels, right along with all those thyroid problems we've already discussed (not a coincidence, incidentally). With 11% of Americans—and one out of four women of childbearing age—on a prescription antidepressant, it's becoming painfully obvious that toxins aren't giving our brains a free pass when it comes to destroying our health.

It'll be no surprise here to find that inflammation is, once again, at the root of the hormonal disruption that can negatively affect brain function. As if the insults to your thyroid and adrenals weren't enough, the brain is another sensitive area that can become damaged by an onslaught of toxins and the stress they induce. And, as we've already seen, these seemingly different systems are all intimately connected so that what affects one system inevitably will affect the other systems of the body. This explains why treating thyroid issues or mental health issues without simultaneously addressing issues in the gut is a recipe for failure.

Numerous studies have illustrated the link between gut health and brain function, demonstrating that inflammatory markers in the blood correlate with the risk for depression.

When inflammation begins in the gut, the immune system produces cytokines—special chemical messengers produced by immune cells in response to pathogens and toxins. As these cytokines travel throughout your body, they eventually can cross the blood-brain barrier and incite inflammation in the brain, leading to depression and other issues with mood, memory, and cognition.

Hormones and other chemicals entering the brain through the bloodstream aren't the only way the gut and brain are connected either. The nervous system plays an important role in communicating between these two organs. Ever had butterflies in your stomach when you felt nervous, or been too stressed to eat? This is your brain and gut talking to each other via the enteric nervous system. The gut is lined with neurons—nerve cells that communicate with the brain via the vagus nerve.

When you're feeling stressed, the activity of the vagus nerve becomes decreased, meaning many of the functions of digestion, such as stomach acid production, enzyme secretion, and rate of digestion are dampened. When stress is chronic, such as when toxins constantly bombard your system, the digestive system and, by association, the brain, takes another hit to optimal functioning.

Back to You, Immune System

All of this stress-induced hormones-run-amuck leads back to one major area that we've only been hinting at up until now: the immune system. Or, more specifically, an immune system that's chronically fired up to the point that it loses sight of its end goal of protecting the body from outside invaders and begins to attack the body itself. We call this type of immune system cannibalism *autoimmunity*. No longer able to differentiate between foreign invader and self, the immune system begins to destroy the very tissues it's meant to protect, leading to full-blown autoimmune disease—from the all-too-common thyroid autoimmune disease to more serious, and life threatening, diseases such as, multiple sclerosis, rheumatoid arthritis, and, even, cancer.

Autoimmunity is the result of an overwhelmed and overworked immune system. No longer able to keep up with the constant flux of toxins filtering in through a leaky gut (which is always a factor in autoimmune disease), toxins pile up as the various systems of the body, from the digestive system to the brain, succumb to the toxic overload and the hormonal chaos that ensues. As this toxic overload builds up year after year, the immune system grows more overwhelmed until it's weakened and confused, attacking anything and everything in sight in a desperate attempt to control the chaos. From the brain to the thyroid, the joints and the adrenals—no part of the body is (pardon the pun) immune.

Why Does the Body Attack Itself?

Researchers into the area of autoimmunity have discovered that three factors are always present in order for autoimmunity to manifest. As we've just mentioned, leaky gut is one of those factors. The second factor is the environmental trigger—the toxins—that goad the immune system into hyperactivity. The third factor is genetics. While leaky gut and toxins are a recipe for autoimmunity, exactly how that autoimmune condition will manifest itself is determined by your genetic makeup. For one person, it could be celiac disease, where gluten (the toxin) damages the gut (leaky gut) and causes the immune system to attack intestinal tissue. For another, it could present as rheumatoid arthritis, wherein the immune system attacks and destroys joint tissues. Still, for others, the immune system may go on to attack nerve tissue, resulting in multiple sclerosis.

There are over 300 diseases classified as autoimmune, some of which may surprise you. Psoriasis, schizophrenia, heart disease, and, even, cancer is now thought to be autoimmune in nature. Not only that, if you have an autoimmune disease, your chances are greatly increased that you will develop a second or third autoimmune disease later on.

Sounds like scary stuff. But, I'm not here to leave you hopeless and afraid that some dreaded disease is waiting just around the corner to take you out. On the contrary, everything we've discussed so far should be very good news, whether you already have an autoimmune disease or you can relate to any of the alarming health issues we've discussed.

Now we know what's at the root of unrelenting fatigue, moodiness, and brain fog. And we know exactly how it's affecting our hormones and our brains. Wouldn't the logical conclusion be to remove the cause of the whole mess in the first place so we can dial down inflammation, calm the immune system, and reset our hormones?

Unfortunately, when women show up to their doctors complaining of the above symptoms, the root cause of inflammation and toxicity is hardly, if ever, addressed. Often, women are sent on their merry way with a prescription for thyroid hormone, an antidepressant, and other pharmaceutical drugs, which only perpetuate the cycle of toxicity and inflammation. Thankfully, there's a better way. And, it's totally within your grasp. Ditching the toxins and healing the gut are the only true solutions to stopping fatigue, depression, and, even, autoimmunity in their tracks.

What are these toxins that are decimating the health of far too many women today, anyways? Why are we being bombarded by toxins at an unprecedented rate today and how can we protect ourselves from the onslaught? We're going to dive right into those nasty toxins and ditch them one by one in the coming chapters.

First, however, let's look at exactly how your body responds to those toxins and works to eliminate them in an important process known as *detoxification*. Once you know exactly how your body works to rid itself of those nasty toxins, you can start working *with* your body to keep it nourished and strong so, when toxins come knocking, your body's own detoxification pathways can usher them right on out the door just like a bouncer at a Hollywood A-lister party.

Chapter 4
Detoxification Demystified

Detoxification. What does the word mean to you? Does it conjure up images of people sweating half their body weight off in a sweat lodge on some detox retreat in the middle of the desert? Does it mean eating nothing but salads and grapefruit or downing raw apple cider vinegar with a whole spoonful of cinnamon? (Side note—please don't try this). Maybe you've read about some of the more interesting methods used to detox, such as coffee enemas, and quickly decided detoxifying wasn't for you.

Let's face it, detox has gotten a bad rap. With detox methods running the gamut, from "the grapefruit diet" to prepackaged detox kits sold at the grocery store that promise to rid your body of toxins and extra pounds, but usually just leave you with a nasty case of diarrhea, it's no wonder many are wary when the term "detoxification" is bandied about.

Before you write off detoxification as some weird, extreme practice, let's take a look at what detoxification truly is: a process that our body goes through every hour of every day to rid itself of unwanted toxins so the body can function optimally.

Detoxification — A Critical Process

Yep, that's right. Every minute of every hour of every day, your body is being assaulted by toxins. They're in the air you breathe, the foods you eat, the miracle cream you rub on your skin each morning, your shampoo, your favorite antibacterial wipes you use to clean your counters, in your couch, your mattress . . . *I could go on.*

While humans are being exposed to toxins at an unprecedented rate, the good news is, your body is equipped to handle these toxins—to a degree. Your body's detoxification pathways are working day and night to rid your body of the toxic buildup it accumulates through your daily interactions with life. Some of these toxins are naturally occurring byproducts of metabolism. As your body moves, thinks, and digests, metabolic waste products are produced. These internal, or endogenous, toxins come with the territory of being human and your body is equipped to efficiently rid itself of these toxins.

External toxins, on the other hand, are those toxins that we are exposed to from the outward environment. These external, or exogenous, toxins include things like heavy metals, industrial pollutants, and, even electromagnetic radiation. These toxins pose a real threat to our health when they become too much for the body to handle. When your body's ability to break down and eliminate toxins becomes overwhelmed, toxins are stored in our fat cells where they interfere with body chemistry, creating inflammation and disrupting hormonal balance.

Take a look at these signs that a toxic environment is depleting your normal health and energy. These signs all point to one thing—difficulty carrying out the normal processes of digestion, elimination, and detoxification:

- Fatigue
- Joint Pain
- Back aches

- Headaches
- Bad breath
- Allergies
- Frequent Colds
- Sinus Problems
- Constipation
- Acne, Eczema and other skin problems
- Depression/Anxiety
- Difficulty Losing Weight

Any of those sound familiar? If you're like most people in our modern society, I'm sure you can relate to at least a few of these signs that it's time to give your detoxification pathways a little love.

Your Body — The Great Detoxifier

As we saw in the last chapter, when your body is functioning at an optimal level of health, your immune system functions optimally as well, identifying and destroying foreign invaders and neutralizing toxins. Your digestive tract assimilates nutrients from your food and flushes out toxins and waste efficiently. The cardiovascular system delivers those nutrients and oxygen to your cells throughout the body, ensuring every tissue and cell is supplied with what it needs to get the job done.

It's a beautiful picture. *When it's functioning properly*. But, when even one link in the chain becomes weak, everything suffers. In fact, while scientists classify our organs into different body systems for the sake of understanding and interpreting their functions, they are all interrelated.

We've already seen how cognitive problems like depression, for example, can have more to do with an imbalance in the gut than the brain. If you're still wondering how that can be the case, just consider the fact that your gut is lined with *neurons*—nerve cells that communicate directly with the brain through the enteric nervous system. Called the "second brain", the gut produces more of the feel-good hormone, *serotonin*, than your brain does and has a very direct impact on your mood and emotions.

And you thought the digestive system only revolved around eating and pooping. Obviously, it pays to have a healthy body that's capable of ridding itself of the toxins that assault us on a daily basis. We've already looked at how leaky gut contributes to fatigue and brain fog. Let's look at how the digestive system plays a role in detoxification as well.

Your Digestive System—An Overview

The digestive process begins in the mouth, with the act of chewing and swallowing food. When we chew our food, the salivary glands in the mouth release enzymes that begin to break down the foods we eat into easy-to-digest particles.

The act of chewing further breaks down the foods we eat so that we can optimally digest the nutrients within them. This is an important point about digestion that many people don't give much thought to in our fast-paced society. By simply taking the time to thoroughly chew your food before swallowing, you'll be improving your digestion and, thus, your ability to utilize the nutrients within the foods you consume. We'll revisit eating habits later on but, for now, just realize that digestion, and thus digestive issues, begin in the mouth.

Once food has been chewed, it passes through the esophagus to the stomach where the process of digestion continues. The stomach is coated with a thick mucus layer to protect the stomach lining from being damaged by stomach acid. Stomach acid is one of the strongest acids around—hydrochloric acid (HCl)—and it's a major player in the digestive process—another piece you may not give much thought to.

For one thing, this strong acid is responsible for breaking down larger proteins into amino acids so they can be absorbed within the small intestine. These amino acids are vital for the growth and repair of tissues, as well as energy production and the function of the immune system. Stomach acid is also responsible for protecting us against foodborne illnesses. This strong acid usually kills off the bacteria and parasites that can lead to food-borne illnesses.

After leaving the stomach, the partially-digested food (now referred to as *chyme*) moves into the small intestine where digestive juices further break down proteins, carbohydrates, and fats into easily assimilated molecules. The liver, gallbladder, and pancreas lend a helping hand at this point as well, secreting their own digestive enzymes and bile into the small intestine. While not considered a digestive enzyme, bile works to break down the fat in the partially-digested food.

By the way, it may be helpful here to define *enzymes*, just so we're clear on the subject. A technical definition would go something like this: a protein produced by a living organism that acts as a catalyst in specific chemical reactions within the body. Since a catalyst speeds up the rate at which a chemical reaction occurs, we can be thankful for those darling little digestive enzymes. Digestion would take a loooong time without them. Which might be OK if you're a sloth. But, I'm guessing you have better things to do than lay around "digesting" all day long. So, in human speak, enzymes break down the foods we consume and help speed up the rate at which we digest our food.

Once enzymes have further broken down food into easily digested pieces, this is where the magic happens. Nutrients are absorbed via the *microvilli* within the wall of the small intestine where they can be assimilated into tissues throughout the body via the cardiovascular system.

If you think of the GI tract as one long tube from mouth to anus, you will realize that everything that passes this way is technically outside the body. Until the food you've eaten has been broken down and absorbed through that oh-so-important gut wall, it's still not a part of you. Have you ever heard the saying, "You are what you eat"? While there is some truth to that, the reality is: *You are what you digest.* There can be a world of difference between the two when you are dealing with leaky gut syndrome.

When Things Go Wrong: Digestive Issues

If you've ever suffered from digestive issues— be it a temporary case of diarrhea or a serious and ongoing disease like irritable bowel syndrome (IBS)—you know how disastrous digestive problems are to your quality of life. Let's walk back through our digestive system again. But, this time, we'll focus on those areas where a breakdown in the system can cause some serious issues for our digestion.

Since digestion begins within the mouth, the way we chew our food can have a major impact on how well we digest. Gulping down your food without taking the time to properly chew means that large particles of food end up in the stomach and, thus, the intestinal tract, and your body is forced to work much harder to break these food particles into digestible pieces. This leads to a host of issues, from upset stomach to inflammation and food sensitivities, when partially digested food particles end up being absorbed through the gut wall.

Remember how stomach acid helped to further break down proteins? When digestion goes wrong in the stomach, it's usually due to a case of low stomach acid. Contrary to popular belief, issues like heartburn and acid indigestion don't stem from an overproduction of stomach acid. Many medications, as well as infections, such as *Helicobacter pylori (H. pylori)* , suppress the body's natural production of acid in the stomach. When stomach acid is dampened—you guessed it— the body has a hard time breaking down food into an easily digestible form. Gulp down your food and have low stomach acid? You've already got two strikes against your digestion.

Remember where the magic happens in your digestive system? Your small intestine is also where it can all fall apart. Since the small intestine is the site of nutrient absorption, problems with digestion here can have major consequences for your health. By now, you know that, if your small intestine can't properly absorb the nutrients, they can't get inside the cells of your body to benefit you. I won't revisit leaky gut syndrome at this point since we've already explored this common issue. Suffice it to say, leaky gut is responsible for most of our modern problems with inflammation and being undernourished.

After your small intestines have absorbed and assimilated nutrients, the waste moves to the large intestine where water and fiber help to bulk up the stool before it's eliminated from the body. Normally, this should be happening regularly, with a bowel movement happening at least once a day. For many people, however, chronic constipation or chronic diarrhea mark their daily elimination habits—and point to further problems with digestion and detoxification.

Chronic constipation, which can result from hormonal issues, such as a sluggish thyroid or a poor diet, can contribute to toxic overload. When toxins in the gut aren't properly eliminated, they can be recycled back into the liver and stored in the fat tissues of the body.

Chronic diarrhea or loose stools, can indicate a serious problem as well. This condition can result from the body attempting to eliminate foods and substances that irritate the gut. Unfortunately, precious nutrients can also get flushed out in the process, leading to nutrient deficiencies. If irregular bowel movements are normal for you, it's a major clue to problems in the gut. Having normal, healthy bowel movements is vital to ditching the toxins.

The Detoxification Process

The process of digestion is both amazing and complex, isn't it? Unfortunately, along with all those nutrients in your food can come a host of toxins as well. Bacteria and parasites, as well as chemicals, like BPA, may have leached into your food from the plastic packing it came wrapped in.

As toxins pass through your digestive system and are absorbed by the bloodstream, they make their way to the liver where they begin the process of being broken down and eliminated from the body—the process of detoxification. As one of the key players in detoxification, the liver is responsible for deciding which compounds are beneficial for the body and then seeing that they are transported to your tissues for use. The liver also determines which compounds are harmful and repackages them for elimination in a three-phase process of detoxification that requires certain key nutrients and enzymes to be carried out successfully.

During *Phase I Detoxification*, the liver produces enzymes which begins neutralizing potentially harmful toxins. While this process is vital to eliminating toxins from the body, it also has the unfortunate side effect of producing *free radicals* which are in and of themselves quite destructive.

You are probably familiar with free radicals—atoms with unpaired electrons that go around stealing electrons from other compounds in an effort to stabilize themselves. This molecular thievery results in cellular damage and accelerates aging.

Antioxidants put a stop to this oxidative process by lending one of their own electrons to the unstable molecule. Antioxidant nutrients like vitamin C and glutathione (the body's master antioxidant) are, therefore, critical to the function of *Phase I Detoxification*, as well as B vitamins, calcium, and certain amino acids.

Phase II is referred to as *Enzymatic Conjugation,* and is critical to preparing toxins for elimination. Here, toxins which were converted from fat soluble to water-soluble molecules during *Phase I,* are now ready to be paired with other water-soluble molecules, which prepares them to be escorted from the body. Essentially, *Phase II Detoxification* involves adding enzymes to our now water-soluble toxins from *Phase I* so that they are less dangerous and can head down the next path, which is the elimination phase.

There are a number of conjugation pathways that can happen during *Phase II* of detoxification, one of which is known as *methylation.* You might have heard of this one if you have dealt with heavy metal toxicity. In this process, a methyl group is attached to a toxin in a sort of tagging system that let's the liver know this molecule needs to be eliminated. Once again, this process relies on certain key nutrients to make things happen. B vitamins and key amino acids, as well as fiber, are needed to keep things, *ahem*, moving.

Finally, in *Phase III*, the *Transport Phase*, toxins are all packaged up and ready to head out of the body. During *Phase III*, toxins are eliminated through two main pathways: the kidneys (urine) and the bile and colon (stool). The important thing to know about *Phase III Detoxification* is that your elimination habits need to be healthy in order for your liver to do its job of ridding the body of toxins. You can "detox" all day long, but, if you're not having regular healthy bowel movements, all those nasty toxins you've worked so hard to get rid of aren't going anywhere. When toxins just sit in the colon without being eliminated, they can be reabsorbed into the bloodstream where they can travel right back to your tissues—and make you even sicker than before.

The takeaway here is that detoxification is happening on a daily basis as you not only eat, but breathe, and absorb toxins through the skin—and without adequate amounts of the proper nutrients, your ability to ditch these toxins can become seriously dampened, leading to the list of symptoms we saw at the beginning of this chapter. Hopefully, you're starting to get a picture of why proper nutrition is so vital to feeling energetic and healthy. You simply can't rid yourself of the onslaught of toxins without it.

Unfortunately, many people go about "detoxing" all wrong—trying to rid their bodies of toxins without making sure to consume adequate amounts of the right nutrients and fiber, not to mention having proper elimination habits. Now you can see why quick fix methods of detoxification don't work. Simply downing some apple cider vinegar or eating nothing but grapefruit won't provide the nutrients you need to move the toxins out. Even the best detox kit on the market can't do much good if the gut isn't healthy to begin with.

Don't Let Toxins Get the Best of You

Remember the iconic scene from *I Love Lucy* where Lucy and Ethel are tasked with packaging chocolates off a conveyor belt? They start off all right, but suddenly, those darned chocolates just keep coming faster and faster until our funny ladies can't keep up, stuffing chocolates down their shirts and under their hats to hide the evidence of their failure. Well, your liver is kind of like that as well. It does its best to keep up with the daily conveyor belt of toxins thrown its way but, when the load becomes too much, well, what's a liver to do? Toxins get transported to your fat cells for storage where they try to hide out.

When it comes to keeping the body's natural detoxification process going strong, think of it as a two-step system. Step one is to avoid the toxins that are derailing your health and damaging the gut. Step two involves eating an anti-inflammatory diet that's high in the nutrients that fuel detoxification. Don't make the mistake of trying to regain your energy and reset your hormones without making sure that both of these steps are in place. Your chances of ditching the toxins that are leaving you exhausted are pretty slim without both pieces of the detoxification puzzle in place.

Think about it this way: What if, instead of keeping our bodies free from the toxins that undermine our health and nourishing ourselves in a way that strengthens the immune system and promotes proper detoxification, we just keep ignoring the signals the body is sending us, loading up daily with toxic foods, toxic chemicals in makeup, and household cleaners, and not taking the time to instill the habits that promote strong, healthy digestion? Those toxins will continue to accumulate and—it may not be today, it may not be tomorrow—but, at some point, just like Lucy and Ethel, the burden will become too much and the symptoms will appear.

Let's be smarter than that. Let's ditch the toxins now and start treating our bodies like the beautiful creations they are, and that are meant to be nourished and cared for in a way that promotes life and health instead of depression and disease. What do you say? Are you ready to start feeling amazing, energetic, and clear-headed? Are you ready to take down the toxins that are trying to take you down? Let's dive right into those areas where toxins are doing their dirty work and start taking back your health.

Chapter 5
Ditch Toxic Foods

Let's begin our takedown of toxins with what you put in your mouth three times or more every day. Let's knock out a major source of toxins that is clearly slowing us down and contributing to all types of illness, including thyroid dysfunction and adrenal fatigue. Let's talk about food.

Toxins in our food come in all forms. Some I've already mentioned, like gluten, but others you may have never heard of, such as phytates, lectins, and difficult-to-digest proteins like casein. That's not to mention those exogenous toxins that can hitch a ride on the foods we eat, such as pesticide residues, heavy metals, and bacterial contamination.

Unfortunately, our modern diet of processed foods also leaves us deficient in the very nutrients that fuel detoxification. The standard American diet is sorely lacking in the antioxidants, B vitamins, and key minerals that support this critical function. This double whammy of toxin-laden and nutrient deficient foods in the modern diet is a recipe for fatigue and brain fog if ever there was one.

While food is meant to heal and restore our bodies, the sad truth is, modern food is often fraught with toxic dangers that can do more harm than good. No need to panic though! By removing the most offending foods from the diet and loading up on the nourishing foods we were *meant* to eat, we can give our beautiful bodies the tools needed to truly look and feel great!

In the next section, we'll explore the top toxic foods in the modern diet and take a closer look at just how these foods damage our health. You may be surprised to learn that some of the very foods you have been told were good for you are anything but. Then, we'll look at just what you should be eating to restore gut health and ensure proper nutrient intake while dialing down inflammation.

Toxic Foods

Grains

One of the biggest toxic offenders in your pantry are grains, especially gluten-containing grains, like wheat and barley. If you've noticed that going gluten free seems to be the hottest dietary fad of the moment, it's not just because women are realizing that passing on the bread basket is good for the waistline. Gluten intolerance is at an all-time high for reasons that many scientists are still speculating about.

Some believe that our problems with wheat today stem from the fact that it's simply not the same wheat grandma ate. Modern wheat has been hybridized (and often genetically modified) to create larger yields, withstand greater amounts of pesticide use, and even increase the amount of gluten in order to create flour that rises better, creating lighter, fluffier breads and baked goods.

While these changes may help food manufacturers increase profits, the consumer isn't so fortunate. Gluten, a protein found in grains such as wheat, barley, and rye, cannot be fully broken down in the gut because we humans lack the necessary enzymes to do so. Partially undigested gluten proteins make their way to the small intestine, interfering with nutrient absorption and triggering intestinal permeability, which we've already learned is a major contributor to thyroid, adrenal, and immune issues.

If you thought a gluten-free diet was only for those who've been diagnosed with celiac disease, think again. Gluten sensitivity is surprisingly common—some researchers even assert that no human can properly digest this difficult protein and signs of intolerance are only a matter of time. Those signs of intolerance, by the way, can be varied and often surprising. Health issues that go way beyond digestive discomfort—joint pain, depression, allergies, skin rashes and dryness are just a few of the over 250 symptoms that have been associated with gluten intolerance. The takeaway here is that no one is immune to the damage gluten does to the gut.

Gluten isn't the only toxin grains bring to the table either. The seeds of grains contain chemical compounds which make them difficult to digest. One of the worst offenders is a class of proteins known as *lectins*. Lectins in grains have a whole host of issues they bring to the gut. Let's look at a few of them.

Lectins are a defense mechanism of seeds and are, thus, very difficult to digest. This difficulty digesting lectins translates into damage to the gut lining—yes, leaky gut strikes again. Remember our lesson on leaky gut? When the tight junctions of the gut wall become overly permeable, anything and everything that enters the digestive tract—bacteria, viruses, undigested food particles—can cross the gut wall and into the body via the bloodstream.

All this gut irritation has the unfortunate side effect of overstimulating the immune system and triggering inflammation. Of course, some degree of permeability in the gut wall is necessary for the digestion of nutrients, but when intestinal permeability increases beyond normal, the body becomes overloaded with toxins. In those of us who already have increased intestinal permeability, lectins contribute to autoimmunity by entering the bloodstream partially digested where they then elicit an immune response from the body.

Normally, the immune system recognizes a foreign invader and quickly works to eliminate it, at which point the immune system can "calm down" again and go back on the defensive for the next time it's needed. For example, when you catch a cold, your immune system goes on the attack, seeking out and destroying the virus causing the illness. Many of your symptoms aren't so much a product of the virus as they are a product of the immune system. When on the attack, inflammation increases and you notice these signs as fever, swelling, and redness, for example (as in that runny, red nose that keeps going like a faucet). Once the threat has been contained, inflammation decreases in the body and you begin to feel like yourself again.

When the immune system is constantly on the offense, however, the inflammatory response stays elevated—often for weeks, months, or years, in the case of an autoimmune health issue. When we eat things like grains on a daily basis, you're giving your immune system a run for its money, day in and day out. In fact, as Dr. Tom O'Bryan, author of *The Autoimmune Solution*, shared with me, the markers for inflammation in the body that are associated with autoimmunity are present in the body *years* before a full-blown autoimmune condition is diagnosed. Grains can be irritating the gut and immune system for years before you even realize the harm they're causing.

You may be feeling a bit puzzled at this point if you've grown up believing whole grains were good for you. I mean, we all learned about the food pyramid in grade school with wholesome whole grains as the base of a healthy diet. (Yes, I realize the food pyramid has gone the way of the dinosaurs by now, but the newest version of the USDA's dietary guidelines are essentially the same—grains, grains, and more grains!) While it's true that grains do have some redeeming qualities, the bad outweighs the good on this one. Before we move on, let's make sure you're crystal clear on why avoiding grains is a great way to heal the gut and regain your health.

There are a lot of arguments out there today on whether or not grains are healthy. While it's true that humans have been consuming grains for thousands of years, there are several reasons why you might want to seriously consider passing on the bread basket permanently. First of all, many proponents of a grain-free diet point out that the grains of today are very different from the grains our ancestors consumed even a few hundred years ago. Hybridization of wheat has been going on for roughly the last thousand years, increasing the protein content (which increases the elasticity of the flour and makes a nice, light, fluffy loaf of bread), while simultaneously decreasing the amount of nutrients. Did you catch that? When we increase the protein content—the same protein that irritates the gut, we also diminish those important nutrients I keep pointing out as so critical to detoxification and immunity.

Need another reason why grains aren't worth your time? With the majority of grains being genetically modified today, the bread we're now eating is even further from the grains of yesteryear than it's ever been. We'll dive into the problem with genetically modified foods in just a bit, so hold onto the thought that grains are one of the most commonly modified foods around. Suffice it to say for now that GMOs (genetically modified organisms) are modified for one main purpose—so they can withstand higher levels of pesticide use; yet another toxin that damages the gut and irritates the immune system.

Finally, the grains we eat today are different from the grains of our ancestors in another major way: the method of preparation. Ancient cultures were more aware than we are today of how eating grains affected their health, probably because they were more sensitive to the nuances of digestion than most people are today (no, diarrhea on a daily basis is not normal!). For this reason, ancient cultures (and many traditional cultures throughout the world today) took special care in the way they prepared grains before consuming them. This mainly boiled down to three different methods of preparation: fermentation, soaking, and sprouting.

What ancient cultures most likely learned from trial and error was, that by properly preparing grains before eating them, they were easier to digest. Soaking, sprouting and/or fermenting grains helps to break down the proteins that are so hard for the body to digest—those nasty lectins we just looked at, as well as other problematic compounds within grains such as phytates, an anti-nutrient that interferes with mineral absorption.

My advice on grains is this: If you are dealing with digestive issues, an autoimmune disease of any kind, or experiencing any type of health issues, including fatigue, I would recommend removing all grains from the diet. Once you have healed the gut and tamped down the autoimmune response, you may be able to add some grains in selectively, especially if they are properly prepared in the ways we discussed: soaking, sprouting, and fermenting. All except gluten-containing grains, that is. Nix them permanently. They aren't serving your health and research has shown they are damaging to the human gut, autoimmune issue or not. Just do it, for the sake of your health, and don't look back.

Vegetable Oils

One class of foods that needs a closer look for its toxic properties is processed vegetable oils, including corn, soy, and canola. The introduction of processed vegetable oils into the diet of modern humans is a story wrought with bad science, biased social policy, and political missteps. I could write a whole book on the problems with seed crop oils (in fact, whole books *have* been written on the subject), but let's just look at a few of the major reasons to avoid vegetables oils in favor of better choices such as olive, avocado, and ghee.

Back when my grandma was a little girl, her home-cooked meals were rounded out with a healthy dose of natural fats which supplied key nutrients such as vitamin D, vitamin A, and vitamin K2 from sources like butter and whole milk (from cows raised on the farm and fed a natural diet), as well as eggs from the backyard chickens, and saturated fats from animal sources (beef, poultry, etc.).

Enter the processed food industry, who discovered that they could make money off of unwitting consumers by producing and selling cheap crop oils like canola, soy, and corn, and convincing those consumers that their products were healthier than their more natural counterparts through clever marketing campaigns. By the 1950s, America's dietary landscape had changed dramatically. Healthy fats were condemned for their high saturated fat content and margarine and processed vegetable oils replaced butter at the dinner table. Rates of heart disease and cancer began to climb as well, but no one seemed to pay much attention to that.

So, what's the big deal with processed seed oils? In a word, *a lot* (ok, two words). The manufacturing process these oils undergo to even be considered edible is enough to completely damage these fats and render any chance they ever had at being healthy to nil. Just hop on over to YouTube and search for "canola oil production" to see what I mean. You'll find that these oils are mixed with chemical solvents, exposed to high heat, and chemically deodorized and bleached in order to produce the product that sits on the grocery store shelf.

Fats, especially polyunsaturated fats like seed oils, are extremely delicate and easily damaged by exposure to light, heat, and chemicals. When these fats are oxidized in the presence of heat, for example, they form free radicals, which cause cellular damage when ingested. *Yummy.* And, we haven't even mentioned trans fats yet—a totally fake (and totally toxic) form of fats where oils, like soy and corn, undergo a chemical process that unnaturally adds a hydrogen atom to a fatty acid molecule in a configuration that is like nothing seen in nature, and thus derails thousands of chemical processes in the body. These toxic fats have been linked to everything from heart disease to cancer. Yet, we're still eating them.

Can I appeal to your sense of logic here? Does it really make sense that, suddenly, the very fats that have allowed humanity to survive and thrive for thousands of years could be the problem? Doesn't something about the fact that these seed oils are highly processed and tainted with toxic chemicals raise a red flag? Well, manufacturers might be able to fool your sense of logic, but they can't fool your cells.

Every cell in your body is protected by a cell membrane called the phospholipid bilayer. Unless you skipped high school biology that day, you'll recall that *lipid* is another word for *fat*. Yep, every cell in your body is protected by a layer that is composed, in part, of fats. The takeaway here: healthy fats equal healthy cell membranes. Damaged, rancid, poor quality fats equal unhealthy cell membranes. And unhealthy cell membranes are much more susceptible to the onslaught of pathogens and toxins—which is why rates of everything from obesity to cancer and heart disease go up dramatically in populations that consume crop seed oils.

GMOs

One of the most alarming categories of toxins in our foods is genetically modified organisms (GMOs) and their intimate link with pesticides. I spoke with Jeffrey Smith and Amy Hart, producers of the documentary *Secret Ingredients* to get their perspective on what women should know about the dangers of GMOs—and what they told me is a message every mom in America needs to hear. In *Secret Ingredients,* Jeffrey and Amy chronicle the story of real American families and how their switch to a GMO-free diet dramatically impacted their health.

It's been estimated that 75 percent of the food in a typical grocery store is genetically modified. While food producers try to promote GMOs as a safe and cost-effective way to provide food for the growing human population, the scientific literature paints a much different picture. Foods are often genetically modified in order to sustain the ever increasing use of pesticides such as Monsanto's famous *Roundup Ready* herbicide.

Glyphosate, the active ingredient in *Roundup* has a long history of controversy. Jeffrey Smith told me of the work of one of the world's foremost independent researchers in the area of GMO research, Dr. Seralini of France. When Dr. Saralini fed rats a GMO diet of corn that had been sprayed with the *Roundup* herbicide, he found that health problems began to surface within a month and that, within two years, the normal lifespan for a rat, the GMO-fed rats had developed multiple massive tumors, damage to their kidneys and pituitary glands and altered hormone levels, as well as suffering an early death.

I hopped over to Dr. Seralini's website after talking to Jeffrey and was greeted with pictures of lab rats sporting huge tumors, piglets with birth defects, and other horrors of GMO exposure—including those to children. If you're brave enough, do your own Google search of Dr. Seralini and his work to see for yourself. GMOs are like a science experiment gone horribly wrong.

Corn and cotton are genetically modified to withstand the use of *Roundup* herbicide. They've also been modified to produce their own insecticide known as *Bt toxin*. Jeffrey

Smith shared with me that this toxin fights insects by "poking holes" in the walls of their intestines, causing them to die when they eat these crops. The companies manufacturing the corn genetically modified to produce Bt toxin have assured the public that these foods are safe for human consumption.

A 2012 study in the *Journal of Applied Toxicology* proves otherwise. This study showed that, in the laboratory setting, Bt toxin pokes holes in human cells as well. By the way, Jeffrey also cited a Canadian study wherein 93 percent of women in the study tested positive for Bt toxin in their blood—and the blood of their unborn fetuses. As Jeffrey Smith pointed out to me, there is no blood-brain barrier in the fetus—meaning Bt toxin has the potential to get into the brain of your unborn baby. Yep, that's right, a hole-poking toxin in the brain of unborn babies.

Finally, Bt toxin has been found to provoke an immune response in humans and animals, even causing sensitivities to formerly harmless substances. This may be one piece of the puzzle to why allergies are on the increase along with all other categories of chronic illness. The bottom line with GMOs is that we're all part of one giant experiment on the outcome of these toxins on human health. Do yourself and your family a favor and avoid GMOs whenever possible by choosing foods labeled as *organic* and *GMO-free*.

I'd also recommend checking out the documentary, *Secret Ingredients*, released January 2017. You can find details of the movie at SecretIngredientsMovie.com. I'm also offering my interview with Jeffrey Smith and Amy Hart as a bonus to this book, which you can find here. I think you'll find it enlightening. I know I certainly did.

Processed Foods

Consuming processed foods may just be one of the top ways we destroy our own health. Not only are these foods chock-full of many of the toxic foods we've already looked at—trans fats, grains, soy additives, GMOs, and sugar—they also come loaded with chemical additives, which have been shown to damage gut health and increase—you guessed it—inflammation. Just take a look at virtually any packaged, processed foods out there and you'll likely see a long list of unpronounceable chemicals. Most of the time, we look at the label, wonder what sodium benzoate, soy lecithin, or monoglycerides really are, then shrug our shoulders and assume that, if it wasn't safe to consume it wouldn't be there . . . right? Wrong. As we've already seen, *dead wrong*.

Just consider artificial food coloring for one. These chemical additives have been linked to impaired behavior in children—and now studies are showing that we're consuming way more than we originally thought we were. Additionally, Dr. Natasha Campbell-McBride, creator of the GAPS diet, shares on her website that artificial colors also have been shown to possess antimicrobial and antifungal properties which damage our delicate gut microbiome. And artificial coloring is just one of the many additives manufacturers put in processed foods to enhance the color, texture, and taste.

I'm sure it's no surprise to see processed foods on the list of most toxic foods for the body. I mean, nobody's making a case for potato chips and ice cream to top the list of healthy foods. Unfortunately, many packaged processed foods have been given a marketing spin to make you think they're healthier than they really are. From "low-fat" to "high-fiber", the dietary pitfalls of these "foods" (I use the term loosely) far outweigh any presumed benefits.

I remember, back in the day, when I thought high-fiber granola bars were healthy and low-fat yogurt was a great snack (despite the 20 plus grams of sugar it contained). One brand of low-fat, high-fiber granola bars was a particular favorite of mine. At the time, I struggled with some annoying—not to mention—embarrassing digestive issues, including gas and bloating. While I was complaining of my digestive woes to my sister one day, she suggested it might be those healthy high-fiber granola bars I was eating *every day*. The idea seemed novel at the time but, when I ditched the granola bars, guess what? No more embarrassing gas and bloating.

It seems bizarre to me now to think that I was so out of touch with how the foods I was consuming were affecting me, but I hadn't yet learned to make the connection. After all, the healthy marketing spin many processed foods are given make it easy to fall for the hype that these artificially flavored, preservative-containing sugar bombs are the answer to eating healthy.

Do yourself a favor and look past all the empty promises on the label of processed foods and, instead, look at the ingredients list. If you see a long list of unpronounceable chemicals and additives, sugar in its various forms (high-fructose corn syrup, maltose, sucrose, etc.), processed seed oils, or nutrient-depleted grains—put it back on the shelf and head for the produce section instead.

Dairy

Let's move on to another toxic food that's damaging to the gut and upping the inflammation in your body. While you might not think of it this way, the vast majority of dairy products available today are really just a subclass of processed foods we looked at as a source of dietary toxins. Yeah, I know the International Dairy Board (or whoever the powers that be in the world of dairy marketing) would have you believe that milk and its ilk are the wholesome, natural products of yesteryear that create strong bones, teeth, and muscles. How can all those celebrities be wrong, with their cute milk mustaches, admonishing us to "*Drink Milk*"?

The thing is, milk can be a healthy source of nutrients, protein, enzymes, and probiotics—*if* it's raw and sourced from healthy animals fed a natural diet. And, that is where conventional dairy products fail the test as a healthy food. Dairy's dirty little secret (which isn't such a secret anymore, thanks to documentaries like *Food, Inc.*) is that modern dairy practices, like pasteurization and homogenization, remove most, if not all, of the nutrients, enzymes, and probiotics that dairy *should* provide.

Pasteurization, the process whereby milk is heated to 161.6 F for 15 seconds, is meant to kill off dangerous bacteria that have the potential to cause serious illness. When this process was invented over 100 years ago, it was thought to be a boon to public health. The chances of contracting serious foodborne illnesses, like listeriosis, were practically eradicated. The unfortunate side effect, however, was the destruction of the beneficial bacteria that help your body digest the fats, proteins, and sugars in milk.

Not only are beneficial microbes lost in the process of pasteurization, but many essential nutrients, such as vitamins A, C, and the B vitamins, are destroyed as well. Pasteurization also destroys valuable enzymes that help our bodies digest milk as well as denaturing proteins. That's a lot of damage to one poor little food source. Unfortunately, dairy manufacturers don't stop there.

Undoubtedly, you've noticed that every gallon of milk you've purchased from the grocery store proudly proclaims "Pasteurized and Homogenized" on the label. For those of us who grew up having never seen milk in its raw form, we might have been surprised as kids by the way raw milk separated from the cream—an inconvenience that, apparently, warranted its own manufacturing process within the food industry.

Homogenization is the process of breaking down the fats in milk into very tiny particles that are then suspended throughout the fluid (instead of rising to the top). Housewives everywhere can be forever thankful that this process has saved them from having to shake the milk before serving it to their thirsty families. Unfortunately, just like many modern processes meant to make our lives easier, the unforeseen side effects may well outweigh the benefits. When milk goes through the homogenization process, the delicate fats are oxidized, damaging them in a way that makes them harmful rather than beneficial—as we've already learned from looking at processed vegetable oils.

The dairy industry, like most industries, is concerned with increasing profit while minimizing operating costs and many of the tactics developed to do this have disastrous effects on the consumer's health. One way to cut costs is to feed dairy cows grains, such as corn or soy, as opposed to allowing them to eat their natural diet of grass. And, that's not the worst of it. In an effort to save money, dairy farmers routinely feed their cows everything from cement kiln dust to cardboard and expired packaged foods (what we would effectively consider garbage). It doesn't take a rocket scientist to know that animals fed this unnatural and unhealthy diet are going to be far from healthy themselves.

What's a dairy farmer to do with all those unhealthy animals if he's hoping to turn a profit? Antibiotics to the rescue! Animals raised on factory farms, whether for meat or milk, are routinely given antibiotics in their feed to keep them alive and healthy—at least healthy enough not to die or sicken the other animals around them. These antibiotics make their way into the milk and meat of these unfortunate animals, where they are then consumed by humans. You can add one more point to the leaky gut scorecard, if you're keeping track.

As you can see from the way commercial milk is processed, it is a far cry from the healthy enzyme and probiotic-rich food that our ancestors once consumed. If you choose to incorporate milk into your diet, I strongly recommend you find a quality source of raw milk from healthy, grass-fed animals.

However, you should be aware that many people cannot tolerate even raw milk in their diet due to food sensitivities or allergies. If you are struggling with thyroid problems or an autoimmune disease and need to heal your gut, most experts recommend avoiding all dairy products. Once the gut has healed, it may be worth experimenting with adding raw dairy back into the diet to see if it is tolerated.

Cultured, raw dairy is thought to be especially beneficial, including raw milk kefir and yogurt.

Healing Foods

After reading through the list of toxic foods we just discussed, I'm guessing you may be feeling one of two things. Either you've already discovered the power that comes with avoiding toxic foods and are feeling empowered to hear that the changes you've made are on the right track—or you are thinking that everything on the list of toxic foods is on your daily menu and you have no idea how you could survive without them.

I know that feeling of overwhelm at learning that some of your favorite foods—some of the foods that you thought were good for you—are actually creating a toxic environment in your body that's contributing to exhaustion and gut problems. So, what *do* you eat? When the majority of foods you consume on a daily basis are suddenly off limits, it's tough.

Let's walk through some of the best foods to restore your body to a state of health and wholeness so you can restore the gut and regain your energy. Thankfully, there are plenty of options that will have you feeling energetic, strong, and satisfied. The good news is, they're delicious as well.

What's The Perfect Diet?

With a new dietary philosophy popping up every year, how do you know which one is the best? Is it South Beach, Paleo, or raw foods? Should you try the Wahls Protocol? The bone broth diet? The truth there is one perfect diet—and there isn't. *Allow me to explain.*

The perfect diet is the diet that has sustained us humans for thousands of years. The foods that have allowed us to grow, reproduce, and produce. This diet consists of **real** food. Food that comes from the land, in its natural form, fresh and minimally processed. The *form* this "perfect diet" takes isn't so much what matters as does the substance.

That's because we are all bio-individual, with unique needs that depend on our stage of life, hormonal nuances, and even our toxic load. Whether you choose to follow a Paleo version of the "perfect" diet or a Mediterranean version isn't the point. As a matter of fact, your dietary needs can change throughout your lifetime. While men often do well on the higher fat ketogenic diet, many women struggle with hormonal issues that accompany carbohydrate restriction. Likewise, protein needs can vary depending on your level of activity and health status. This is why subscribing to one specific "diet" can be detrimental to your health. If it's the wrong diet for you, you won't thrive on it.

However, there are some basic tenets the above mentioned diets all hold in common. They all generally ascribe to a way of eating that eschews processed foods, including the toxic foods we looked at above. They recommend plenty of high quality foods that are nutrient-dense and probiotic-rich. Foods that come in their most natural, whole state, as we'll see in a moment.

I would, however, caution against subscribing to a vegan diet. While it may be beneficial in the very short term—for someone dealing with a serious health condition, such as cancer, for example—a vegan diet lacks many of the essential nutrients that are vital to good health, such as vitamin B12. I've heard many a story of the person who develops serious health issues within a few years of going vegan. Much of that is likely due to the fact that grains and processed soy products make a regular appearance on a vegan menu and we've already discussed the problems with these foods. I strongly recommend incorporating some healthy animal products into your diet in addition to the other foods we'll look at below.

So, what are those foods that have nourished humans for the past millennia? Getting plenty of these foods ensures adequate amounts of those nutrients that fuel detoxification and strengthen the immune system. Take a look at the list of healing foods that follows and be sure to incorporate as much of these foods into your daily diet as possible.

Real, Whole Foods

Since we discussed the dangers processed foods pose to your health, it should be no surprise that real, whole foods are just what's on the menu. The closer to their natural state these foods are, the better. Look for fruits and vegetables that are organic, non-GMO, and grown locally, whenever possible (including your own backyard if you have the time and inclination).

When it comes to vegetables, the sky's the limit, from asparagus to zucchini. Green, leafy veggies, dark colored fruits and vegetables, and cruciferous veggies, such as broccoli and cabbage, are some of the best choices. I can't sing the praises of the healing power of plant foods enough—and, if you get enough of them in your diet, you will too. Rich in antioxidants, trace minerals, bioflavonoids, enzymes, and even probiotics from the soil, plant foods are chock-full of the energy producing nutrients we humans need to thrive.

Just consider lycopene, a carotenoid that gives tomatoes their bright red color. Studies have shown that lycopene acts as a powerful antioxidant and has been beneficial in preventing those dreaded inflammatory diseases we all want to avoid: heart disease, Alzheimer's, and cancer. Polyphenols are yet another class of phytochemicals that are powerful antioxidants found in foods like tea, wine, chocolate, and olive oil, as well as fruits and vegetables. Just like their kissing cousins, the carotenoids, polyphenols are known for their disease fighting abilities and can protect the heart, lungs, brain, and other organs from disease.

Or consider curcumin, a polyphenol found in turmeric. I wouldn't be surprised if you've been hearing about the health benefits of turmeric in the news lately. That's because study after study has shown curcumin to be a highly powerful anti-inflammatory, outperforming prescription pharmaceuticals with their ability to combat pain as well as diseases, such as Alzheimer's and even cancer. It's impossible to overestimate the power of food to restore and nourish our bodies.

Make sure to get in as many servings of vegetables each day as you can. Research has shown that most of us aren't eating nearly enough of the green stuff. Try adding a green smoothie to your morning routine, or a salad with lunch. Soups made from homemade bone broth, quality protein, and plenty of vegetables (with a drizzle of good quality olive oil on top) is just about the perfect meal, in my opinion.

Fruits can also be a great way to get many nutrients and enzymes into the body, but, because of their higher sugar content, you will want to limit your consumption of fruit to a few pieces a day and stick to fruits that are lower in sugar, especially while working to heal the gut and restore hormonal balance. Berries, such as blueberries, cherries, and blackberries are a good choice because of their high antioxidant content. Green apples are another good choice. Again, it's best to choose fruits that are grown locally and seasonally, whenever possible. If you struggle with thyroid problems that leave you feeling cold much of the time you may find it difficult to consume much fruit in the winter. Fruit has a cooling effect on the body and is best eaten in season. One option for winter is to consume fruits cooked, such as baked apples or a grain-free blueberry crisp straight from the oven.

High Quality Protein

Toxins tend to accumulate as they move up the food chain, which means we need to be especially careful with the quality of animal protein we consume. Just like the problems with consuming conventional dairy products, many of the same issues apply to meat as well. Conventionally raised meats are fraught with hormones, antibiotics, and other toxins. Just like dairy cows, cattle raised for beef on factory farms are fed an unnatural diet of grains (and other things) that completely change the nutrient profile of the meat.

When choosing animal proteins to incorporate into your diet, look for meat that is labeled *organic* and *grass-fed*. The good news is that you can often find grass-fed beef in your local grocery store. However, it's a great idea to purchase meat directly from a local rancher to ensure high quality and locally sourced meat. Because grass-fed beef has been fed a natural diet, raised in its natural (low stress) environment, this meat has many advantages over conventional meat where your health is concerned.

For instance, a study conducted by the University of California found that grass-fed beef contains two to three times more *conjugated linoleic acid* (CLA) than conventional beef. CLA is a type of fatty acid that is known to protect against inflammation and cancer. Not only are levels of CLA higher in grass-fed cows, many other nutrients and minerals are higher as well, including zinc, calcium, and vitamin A, to name a few. When choosing meat, I urge you to choose carefully and look for grass-fed beef, bison, and other ruminant animals, whenever possible.

Poultry is another animal protein subject to the same sad fate as red meat. Conventionally raised poultry are often fed an unnatural diet high in GMO grains. When choosing poultry for your dinner table, look for organic, free-range chicken and turkey. Your local poultry farmer is a great place to start. The same goes for eggs, by the way. If you can find eggs from free range, organic chickens, it will be worth the money. You can find local, grass-fed beef, free-range poultry, and farm fresh eggs near you at *eatwild.com*.

Finally, seafood is another great choice for getting quality protein in your diet—if you choose carefully. Much of the seafood on the market today is farm-raised and, again, fed an unnatural diet that interferes with the nutrient profile of the food. Farmed salmon is often dyed with food coloring to give it a "natural" pink coloring you would find in wild salmon. When purchasing seafood, it's best to look for wild caught fish, such as wild caught salmon or tuna.

Be careful when consuming predatory fish, however. As already mentioned, toxins tend to accumulate as they move up the food chain and this is especially problematic in seafood because of the high mercury content. Fish, like tuna and swordfish, are best eaten only occasionally in order to avoid mercury—a serious toxin we'll look at more closely in an upcoming chapter. Personally, I look for wild caught salmon, sardines, or whitefish and stick with brands such as Wild Planet for canned seafood. Vital Choice is another great option for finding high quality seafood. You can order online at *vitalchoice.com*.

High Quality Fats

Sadly, we've been fed a load of BS the size of Texas when it comes to the subject of fats and your health. The low-fat craze of the '80s and '90s may well have been one of the darkest hours for our nation, nutritionally speaking. Even though much of the misunderstanding about fats has been proven wrong the myths still abound. Recently, I had to make a trip to my local county health department. I cringed to see posters covering the walls encouraging parents to feed their kids skim milk (other problems with milk aside) as well as lean meats.

The truth is, despite our low-fat diets, health issues, like heart disease, obesity, and cancer (the very diseases low-fat diets are supposed to protect us from) have skyrocketed. Somewhere in the midst of our dietary flogging of natural healthy fats, like those in grass-fed beef and other whole unprocessed foods, such as avocados and egg yolks, another kind of fat was championed as healthier for your heart and body—vegetable oils. We've already explored the host of problems associated with consuming vegetable oils and, hopefully by now, you're convinced that avoiding them is one of the best things you can do for your health.

Since processed vegetable oils are off the table when it comes to a healing diet, does that mean all fats are bad for you? Absolutely not! Natural, healthy fats from whole foods are some of the densest sources of nutrients around. Let's take a look at some of the best.

Avocados are a great source of plant-based monounsaturated fats in addition to a whole slew of minerals and antioxidants. The fat in avocados helps your body absorb nutrients, such as vitamin A and vitamin E. There are several fat-soluble vitamins, by the way, that can only be properly absorbed in the presence of fats—which is one of the many reasons why a low-fat diet is so problematic. So, don't be shy! Eat up those healthy fats and your body will thank you.

Coconut oil is another plant-based source of fat you've probably been hearing a lot about lately. Once shunned for its high saturated fat content, coconut oil is getting its day in the sun. Coconut oil is composed of three main types of medium-chain fatty acids that each bring some unique healing properties to your plate.

One type of fatty acid found in coconut oil is lauric acid. Prized for its antibacterial and antifungal properties, lauric acid helps to balance the gut microbiome, making it an especially great choice to incorporate into the diet while detoxing.

A word on choosing coconut oil. At this point, it probably won't surprise you to learn that coconut oil, like most other foods on the market today, can be heavily processed, decreasing its nutritional benefits. When shopping for coconut oil, look for extra-virgin coconut oil from a sustainable source.

Ghee is one of my favorite fats to consume, and not just because it tastes delicious. Ghee is a nutritional powerhouse loaded with fat-soluble vitamins and healthy saturated fats. If you're not familiar with ghee, it's simply butter that has been simmered until the milk solids rise to the top where they are then skimmed off, leaving the pure butter fat. Because the milk solids have been removed, ghee is free of casein and lactose—two components of milk that are responsible for allergies and sensitivities.

Ghee is chock-full of those fat-soluble vitamins I've been trumpeting throughout this chapter, especially vitamin A, vitamin D, and (one of my favorite vitamins) vitamin K2. Oh, and remember that heart healthy conjugated linoleic acid (CLA) you can find in grass-fed beef? Ghee from grass-fed animals is also a great source of CLA.

Extra-virgin olive oil has a wealth of benefits, including natural phenols, whose anti-inflammatory nature will help dial down an overactive immune system. I like to save olive oil for dressing salads or adding a splash to a stir-fry since excessive heat can be damaging to the easily-oxidized fatty acids in this oil. A word of caution when purchasing olive oil: quality is important. Many of your common grocery store brands of olive oil are actually mixed with cheaper seed oils like soybean oil (yes, even though the label says it's 100% pure extra virgin olive oil). Just one more place where your friendly neighborhood food manufacturer likes to stick it to you. But, I digress.

One brand of olive oil I would highly recommend is Kasandrinos Greek Olive Oil. I've used it for years and have loved the quality of the olive oil as well as the passion for quality that the owners have for their product. You can shop for Kasandrinos oil here. I've also ordered olive oil from Thrive Market, which I've found to be of excellent quality as well.

In fact, I get most of my high quality fats— ghee, coconut oil, and tallow from Thrive Market, as well as many other foods, like canned salmon and real salt. Thrive Market works like a wholesale buying club for organic and natural foods—think Costco, only online. I've found that they have excellent prices and great customer service. You can give Thrive Market a try at http://thrv.me/8ymhJP.

Fermented Foods

If gut health is the hottest topic in the world of medicine these days, then fermented foods are probably the most talked about in the nutrition world as well. These probiotic rich foods, including sauerkraut, kimchi, kombucha, and kefir, help to repopulate the gut with healthy bacteria and restore balance to the microbiome.

The bacterial strains in fermented foods have been shown to break down and neutralize many of the toxins we ingest, including pesticides and heavy metals. By breaking down these toxins before you have had a chance to even consume them, probiotic foods lighten your toxic load while providing key nutrients and, of course, beneficial gut bacteria as well. Talk about a win-win!

These beneficial bacteria can also synthesize important nutrients in the gut, including certain B vitamins and vitamin K—and we now know how vital these nutrients are to the detoxification process. You can thank your beneficial gut bacteria for helping ensure you have plenty of these vital nutrients around to keep you healthy and your immune system going strong.

Fermented dairy products, such as yogurt, kefir, and raw cheese are a great way to get fermented foods into your diet. Just be aware that the same problems with dairy we've already discussed can be a factor in fermented dairy products as well. Most yogurts, kefir, and cheese on the market today are made from conventional dairy—antibiotics, hormones, and other insidious farming practices included. The milk used to make yogurt is usually pasteurized as well, which kills off the beneficial bacteria. The strains of bacteria are added back in after the milk has been "cultured" so, I would argue that what you are getting is not a true fermented food.

Remember to start with raw dairy from healthy cows to make your fermented dairy products. Many people who cannot tolerate even high quality raw milk may be able to consume raw milk kefir and yogurt. Studies have shown, that those who are lactose intolerant have been able to drink raw kefir without issue. If you still find dairy to be a problem for you, you can find coconut kefir and yogurt made from coconut milk.

Fermented vegetables are a great choice for everyone, including kids. Fermented veggies can be simple and inexpensive to make at home. Sauerkraut is a great fermented food to start with when you begin experimenting with fermenting foods.

If you're new to fermented foods, I would recommend checking out Cultures for Health—they have free ebooks and video tutorials, as well as supplies for getting started making your own home ferments. You can visit their website at *culturesforhealth.com*.

Before we move on to the next area of toxins, let's recap. By ditching the toxic foods that damage the gut and derail your energy, and choosing food in their natural, unprocessed and uncontaminated forms, you'll not only be giving your gut some major love, your thyroid, brain, and adrenals will thank you as well. Removing the toxins in the other four areas we're about to look at can be critical, but starting with your diet may just be the most instrumental piece in resetting your hormones and regaining your energy.

Because ditching the toxic foods and knowing what to eat instead can be a bit overwhelming, I've created my *Energy Reset Diet: Quick Start Guide,* which you can also download in the bonuses section of this book by clicking here. This guide will take the guesswork out of knowing what foods to eat for energy—and which to avoid.

Chapter 6
Ditch Toxic Chemicals

Each day we are assaulted with a barrage of toxic chemicals that disrupt our delicate hormonal balance and create an inflammatory response within the body. From the chemicals we have no control over—such as those we breathe while sitting in traffic or at the office—to the chemicals we unwittingly, yet deliberately, put on our bodies in the form of skincare and makeup—humanity is experiencing a toxic burden like never before.

Just look at a few of these statistics to get a feel for how many toxins are being ingested daily by the average American:

- There are over 80,000 chemicals on the market today—many of which have **never been tested** for human safety or efficacy.
- In the past 20 years, the European Union has banned over 1,300 chemicals

due to their concerns for safety. In the same time, **the U.S. has banned just 11.**

- Toxins known to cause cancer and interfere with normal development have been **found in human breast milk.**

Truth be told, some of those statistics can sound pretty scary. My purpose in sharing this information is never to create fear, but rather to inform so that we can better protect ourselves and reduce the toxic burden where it's possible so the body can do its job more efficiently when it comes to dealing with those toxins we can't control—unless you can afford to move to a deserted tropical island and lie on the beach all day, away from civilization. If that's the case, congratulations (can I come visit?).

For the rest of us, we are here to take our place in the real world. So, let's step up to the plate and protect ourselves and our families so that we can live the lives we were meant to— healthy, strong, and perfectly capable of dealing with the toxins coming our way—

without adding to the burden by our poor choices. Let's look at a few of the major areas where toxic chemicals attack so we can be well prepared to take them down!

Is Your Skin Care Making You Sick?

Many of us have a toxic relationship with our skincare products. We buy into the hype that purchasing the next "all natural", anti-aging miracle cream will truly erase the years from our face, put an end to our adult acne, and leave us with soft, supple skin that's smoother than a baby's bottom. First, stop and ask yourself if any of the products you've used have truly delivered on those promises. They might seem to work for a while but, far too often, we find ourselves back to square one before long, dealing with the same skin problems that have plagued us for years, sometimes even decades. Yet, we really want to believe that the glowing, healthy skin we crave is just one more product away from being reality. So, we keep getting back on the skincare product merry-go-round, never stopping to question what's going on.

Skincare companies really know how to exploit our weakness for quick fix skin solutions. Promising that all your dreams will come true if you use *their* product to achieve perfect skin, they fail to mention that many of the ingredients in those products create a whole host of problems at the cellular level.

Many chemicals used in skincare products and makeup are known carcinogens, endocrine disruptors, and neurotoxins. Yep, that's right—they're *known* to create these problems in your body. In other words, lab tests have *proven* their toxicity.

Yet, skincare companies don't want to burden you down with this inconvenient information. So, instead, they throw up their smokescreen of beautiful supermodels looking glamorous, slathering beauty products on their pretty faces, and, suddenly, you don't care if those skincare products are made with battery acid—you just want to look like *that*.

We've all been there, so no judging, but once you know the truth, I hope you'll stop being a victim to slick advertising campaigns and start paying attention to what you're really doing to your skin. Knowledge really is *power* and, as we look at some of the worst toxins in our skincare and makeup, I want you to be empowered to make better choices for your health.

I spoke with Trina Felber, founder of the all-natural skincare line, Primal Life Organics, and author of the international bestseller, *Beauty's Dirty Secret,* to get her take on which toxins in conventional skincare products are most likely to wreck our hormones and energy. The following are some of the top toxins on Trina's list of offenders.

The Skin Offenders

Fragrance

This commonly listed ingredient is really just a slew of toxic chemicals. There are up to 35,000 different chemicals that can be combined to create a "fragrance". The danger here is that we really have no idea what chemicals make up a fragrance in a product. Since fragrance is considered a trade secret within the beauty industry, companies are not required to disclose which toxic chemicals they have put in their products under the label "fragrance."

\Not only are many of these chemicals neurotoxins, carcinogens, and endocrine disruptors, they can often be allergenic, causing a reaction in many people.

The Environmental Working Groups, *Campaign for Safe Cosmetics*, released a 44-page report titled, *The Health Risk of Secret Chemicals in Fragrance,* in May 2010, which outlined the dangers associated with the toxic chemicals that are simply labeled as "fragrance" on beauty products. While fragrance is found in virtually every product from lotions to baby wipes, they specifically examined a handful of popular perfume and cologne products.

Of the 17 brand name fragrances they tested, they found 38 secret chemicals not listed on the labels, with the average product containing 14 unlisted chemicals. Per the report, many of these chemicals have never been assessed for human safety, and the results of the ones that have been tested aren't too comforting, having a track record of hormone disruption, cancer promotion, and chemical sensitization.

One of the top concerns with fragrance mentioned in the report included the use of sensitizing chemicals, known for their ability to cause an allergic reaction, leading to conditions such as dry, itchy skin and fragrance-induced dermatitis. Unfortunately, it would be almost impossible to pinpoint which chemical in this toxic sludge is responsible for the reaction since it may or may not be disclosed on the label, meaning you would be powerless to avoid it in the future.

Don't be fooled into thinking that products labeled "fragrance-free" are any better, by the way. This label simply means that the product has been deodorized with chemicals—but not truly free of "fragrance". The chemical goop that makes up this product would have an unpleasant smell, so manufacturers use the very same chemical fragrances that mask the smell of the product and appear to make it odorless. Take my advice and steer clear of any products that list "fragrance" on the label.

Parabens

You'll recognize this class of toxins on your product's ingredients label by their code names—butylparaben, methylparaben, and propylparaben. Used as a preservative to keep bacteria at bay, parabens have the unfortunate side effect of disrupting hormones, contributing to cancer, and reproductive issues. In fact, a whole slew of studies has been conducted on parabens and their ill effect on health.

Parabens do their dirty work by acting as estrogen mimickers within the body. As parabens enter the bloodstream through the skin, they are mistaken for estrogen, which can lead to early onset of puberty in children, reproductive issues, and cancer. One scary side effect of parabens is their ability to cause damage to skin cells in the presence of UV light. Translation: When you slather paraben-containing lotions on your skin, and then step out in the sun, you significantly increase your chance of skin cancer. Studies have even linked the use of parabens, along with other estrogen mimickers, to the potential development of malignant melanoma.

Because of the known dangers of parabens, many products are now labeled as *paraben-free*. But, many products are still using parabens as a cheap and easy way to keep their products from spoiling, despite the known dangers to consumers' health.

Phthalates

A particularly harmful class of toxins, phthalates are also particularly common in skincare and cosmetics. Besides being found in skincare products such as perfumes, moisturizers, eyeshadow, and liquid soaps, phthalates are used in a wide range of other products as well. Phthalates have a jack-of-all-trades ability to perform many roles in various industrial uses and products. Their ability to make plastic products more flexible, as well as to act as a gelling agent, lubricant, and stabilizer, means you can find these toxic chemicals in everything from pharmaceuticals to shower curtains. Quite literally, phthalates are everywhere. The ubiquitous use of phthalates in our society means we are constantly exposed to low levels of these toxins daily. This is alarming because the damage these toxins can do is so insidious—and so well known—that even the government has begun to sit up and take notice.

In 2003, the Centers for Disease Control (CDC) recommended phthalates be studied further to assess their safety for humans. The results were not good. Since the time of the CDC's recommendation, studies have linked phthalates with asthma, autism, breast cancer, and reproductive issues—just to name a few. So dangerous were phthalates found to be, that the Consumer Products Safety Improvement Act, passed in 2008, banned phthalates from use in children's products and also placed an interim ban on some classes of phthalates—but not all. Especially troublesome is the fact that phthalates are not listed on the ingredients label of most products, making it impossible to know when and how much you are consuming.

While it may be next to impossible at this point to avoid phthalates in today's world, you can arm yourself with knowledge of which products are most likely to use phthalates and avoid them. Until phthalates are banned for good, there are a few things you can do to avoid the worst offenders. Avoiding products that contain the generic ingredient "fragrance" on the label is one good place to start.

Another way to avoid phthalates includes avoiding food products packaged in plastic and opting for organic products packaged in glass. Specifically, I'm thinking of milk, which happens to be one of the major sources of phthalates in the American diet. Yes, that's right. You are consuming phthalates with every bite (or drink) when you eat foods that have been packaged in plastic. Plastics used in the milking process, as well as the plastic jugs milk is packaged in, makes it particularly prone to high levels of phthalates—just one more reason to avoid conventional dairy products besides the ones we discussed in the last chapter. Finally, avoid products, both food and skincare, that are packaged in "recycling-code-3" packaging and choose products labeled as "phthalate free" whenever possible to avoid unnecessary exposure to phthalates.

Water

Surprised to see water on the list of toxins commonly found in skincare products? Frankly, I was too. Water is the first ingredient on the list of virtually every skincare product out there. And that's what makes it so dangerous as a toxin. As Trina Felber explained to me, water in these products is usually not purified water—it's straight up tap water. All the toxins commonly found in municipal water are transferred straight into your skin—from heavy metals to chlorine, which dries the skin and interferes with thyroid function. When these toxins are in virtually every product you put on your body, you're getting a hefty dose of them each time you apply and reapply your makeup and skincare products.

Trina went on to explain that pollutants in the water weren't the only strike against this common ingredient either. Water is commonly found listed first on the ingredients label of skincare products, meaning that it's the most abundant ingredient in the product. As a matter of fact, a product can be *up to 95 percent water*, with the other "active" and filler ingredients making up just 5 percent of the product combined. So, besides the fact that you are paying top dollar for products that are mostly just unfiltered tap water, you're also putting an ingredient on your skin that is dehydrating. As the water in these products evaporates, it pulls moisture from the skin, leaving your skin drier than a desert on a hot July day.

While this list may feel daunting, it's just the tip of the iceberg when it comes to toxins commonly found in skincare and cosmetics. However, "knowledge is power" so, now that you know, head to your bathroom and start looking at your beauty and skincare products. See a whole laundry list of unpronounceable chemicals on the products lining your bathroom shelf? No worries, I've got some simple solutions to toxic skincare.

Safe Skin Solutions

The good news here is that you have complete control of what you put on your body in the form of makeup and skincare products. While some of the toxins we've looked at so far are extremely common in today's world of beauty and skincare, you can take heart in knowing that the tide is turning. Many companies are sitting up and taking notice of the fact that consumers no longer want to slather toxins on their skin in the name of beauty. Choosing safe and effective beauty products has never been easier.

DIY Skincare

One great way to make sure that your skincare products contain only the purest and most nourishing ingredients is to make them yourself! If you are a true DIYer and want to explore this option, you can find many recipes in books and online at sites like *Pinterest*.

If mixing ingredients together like a mad scientist sounds a little daunting to you, there's no need to sweat. DIY can be as simple as adding a drop or two of pure essential oils to your favorite carrier oil and applying it to your skin. Lately, I've been using pure jojoba oil to apply to my face and body when I step out of the shower to keep my skin moisturized. Used for thousands of years as a beauty treatment, jojoba oil may not come with the fancy marketing promises that conventional cosmetics do, but I guarantee it works better— and without the toxic side effects of those conventional products.

Coconut oil can be another great oil to use to moisturize your skin as well. Experiment. Find what works best with your skin and, then, take heart that you're a smart consumer who is no longer duped by marketing jargon while you pocket the extra cash you saved buying overpriced skin creams that don't deliver.

And speaking of essential oils, they are a great alternative to many of the toxic chemicals in skincare products. Interestingly, essential oils have been found to have a synergistic effect on the endocrine and immune systems, supporting our body's functions rather than working against them as we've learned synthetic chemicals do. That's not to mention that essential oils are antimicrobial, destroying dangerous bacteria without harming your microbiome. Finally, essential oils have been shown to have a powerful effect on mental health, with many oils being stimulating and energizing.

Toxin Free Beauty

Rather than spend hours scouring the shelves at your local drugstore hoping to find that rare beauty product that isn't loaded with toxins, I like to take the guesswork out of the process. I've included a few of my favorite companies that create pure, wholesome skincare products. These are the products that I personally use and trust to keep myself and my family looking good without the toxins.

Primal Life Organics

I not only love the products Primal Life Organics (PLO) offers, I love their commitment to consumer safety and transparency. PLO founder, Trina Felber, never questioned the safety of the products she applied to her skin until she became pregnant. As a Certified Registered Nurse Anesthetist (CRNA), Trina was more knowledgeable than most on how chemicals are metabolized within the body—and how the wrong chemicals can have a very toxic effect on our bodies. Trina realized the cheap, toxic chemicals that make up most skincare products were not only *not* working, they were causing more harm than good. With a growing fetus to protect, Trina decided to ditch the toxic skincare and create her own line of truly natural products, using food sources to nourish the skin on the cellular level.

Thankfully, for the rest of us, Trina decided to share her amazing products with the world. Using ingredients like organic avocado oil, pure essential oils, and bentonite clay, the basic premise of Primal Life Organics is: *If you wouldn't eat it, don't put it on your skin.* PLO has quickly become one of my favorite skincare lines, not only for the amazing skin care products that deliver true results, but also because of the passion for health, wellness, and toxin free living that Trina and the entire PLO team share. You can find Primal Life Organics products online at PrimalLifeOrganics.com. In the bonuses section of this book you will also find an exclusive coupon code you can use to save on your first order.

BeautyCounter

A cosmetics and skincare company with a serious mission, BeautyCounter was founded by Gregg Renfrew with the intent of offering skincare products you could feel good about putting on yourself and your family. Gregg was your average working mother, never questioning the safety of the products she slathered on herself and her kids, assuming that those lotions and potions at the cosmetics counter *had* to be safe. Learning the truth about the toxins in conventional products changed everything for Gregg.

Determined to offer consumers a product they could truly feel safe applying to their skin, BeautyCounter was born. Armed with a list of over 1,500 toxic chemicals that BeautyCounter commits to never using in their products, their skincare and cosmetics are as powerful and effective as any toxin-laden product you can find. Read more about BeautyCounter's mission and try out their great products online at *BeautyCounter.com*.

W3LL People

W3LL People is yet another great company offering toxin free skincare and cosmetics. I really like the well-rounded selection of cosmetics offered by this company. From concealer to bronzing powders and even liquid eyeliner, W3LL People has got a lot to offer— and won't leave you missing your old toxic products. They offer mini versions of many of their products so you can try them out without emptying your wallet. Shop for W3LL People products at *w3llpeople.com*.

Morrocco Method

Morrocco Method (MM) is a line of hair care products that are unlike anything you've ever tried. Made only from the purest ingredients, these products are safe enough to eat—not that I'm recommending that, of course. Morrocco Method hair care products are truly different than other hair care products out there. This is one company that takes the quality of their ingredients very seriously, not just looking to avoid toxic ingredients, but seeking out only those ingredients that nourish, detoxify, and feed the scalp and hair with each use.

A word to the wise on how to use these products: Because MM is truly "natural" hair care, it's very different than your traditional shampoos and conditioners. Don't expect these products to lather, for instance. Fortunately, the company provides plenty of education on their website on how to use their products, including how to detoxify your hair from your conventional products that have built up on your hair and scalp. Be forewarned that the learning curve can be a little tough for some people, but it's totally worth it. The detox process can last up to a few months, but after using MM for a year now, I can attest that my naturally curly hair has never looked better. Shop for Morrocco Method products at MorroccoMethod.com.

Clean With Care

Whew! That's a lot of toxins we just unloaded from our bodies right there! Feels good, doesn't it? We're still not done though—toxins in cleaning products can also build up in our systems as well when we encounter them.

Just like with skincare products, the good news is that safe, effective alternatives to toxic cleaning and laundry products are widely available and more are hitting the shelves every day. This new demand for non-toxic cleaning products means that they are becoming more affordable than ever. Having to DIY all your cleaning products to make sure they are toxin free is a thing of the past. Of course, for those who are true DIYers, it's easier than ever to create your own toxin free cleaning products as well.

Many of the top toxins in cleaning products are the same ones that are in beauty products—phthalates, parabens, synthetic fragrances, and more. Rather than re-invent the wheel, in this section I'm going to offer some of my top picks for toxin free cleaning products as well as super simple ways to DIY, if you want to go that route.

It's truly exciting to see the number of companies on the market today offering products that are free of toxins, environmentally-friendly and socially responsible. Here are just a few of the products I've tried and love. Feel free to try them out or do your own research and find a company you love!

Norwex

Norwex offers chemical free alternatives to cleaning. Emphasis on the words *chemical free*. The star player in their lineup is a high-quality microfiber cloth that can clean just about anything—using only water. When I say high quality microfiber, I'm not kidding— Norwex's microfiber is 1/200th the size of a human hair and contains more than 10 million feet of fiber in just one cloth! This unique design of Norwex microfiber creates a negative chemical charge that attracts dust particles like, well, a magnet. This isn't the typical microfiber you find for sale in the grocery store checkout lane.

Norwex goes way beyond microfiber by the way, including enzyme-based cleansers such as a mattress cleaner and a grill cleaner. Norwex is a direct-sale company, meaning you'll need to find a consultant to purchase products through. You can check out their products and find a consultant in your area at www.Norwex.com. They also offer a line of toxin free skincare products worth checking out.

The Honest Company

If you really love the squeaky clean feel that soap-based products give you, The Honest Company (THC) has a broad range of products for cleaning, laundry, and personal care products. Founded by actress Jessica Alba in 2011 after the birth of her first child, Alba was determined to create an alternative to the toxin-laden baby care products that saturated the market at the time. The Honest Company might be especially exciting to you if you're a momma with a baby—from diapers and formula to baby soap and lotion, THC has everything you need to take care of your little one toxin free. While you can find The Honest Company products at your local Whole Foods and Target stores, you can order online at *www.honest.com* as well.

Mrs. Meyer's Clean Day

Another company I use and love is Mrs. Meyer's Clean Day. Made from plant-based, naturally derived ingredients, these products are safe for the environment and your family. This is another company that has a wide array of cleaning products. I especially like their dish soap scented with pure essential oils instead of those pesky synthetic fragrances we know are so damaging to human health. You can find Mrs. Meyer's products in your local health food or grocery store or order online from Thrive Market.

Is Your Water Toxic?

I recently chatted with Dr. Tom O'Bryan, a leading expert in autoimmunity and author of

The Autoimmune Fix. He explained to me that it's often the little things that can have the biggest impact on our health. For example, he pointed out that the chemical smell of gasoline you inhale every time you fill your gas tank is actually the toxic chemical *benzene*—and you're getting a hefty dose of this carcinogen every time you stop for gas. His solution? Simply walk over to the other side of your car while you're waiting for the gas tank to fill and avoid unnecessary exposure.

The shower is yet one more place where you are absorbing toxins. As you shower, chlorine in the water is absorbed into the skin where it makes it's way to the bloodstream, and from there interferes with the body's ability to utilize thyroid hormone. Again, Dr. O'Bryan emphasized a simple solution. Purchase an inexpensive shower filter to drastically cut down on the amount of chlorine you're exposed to daily. A good quality filter for the kitchen tap is invaluable as well, removing not only chlorine, but other toxic compounds such as heavy metals.

To Dr. O'Bryan's advice I would also add this: avoid drinking from plastic water bottles at all costs. Often, the bottled water on the market is simply tap water and often unfiltered. The real issue with bottled water, however, has to do more with the bottles than the water. The plastics used to make the bottles leach chemicals into the water and the longer it sits—whether in a storehouse somewhere awaiting shipment to the market or on your kitchen shelf—the higher potential there is for plastic to leach into the water, and then into you when you drink it.

I always take a glass water bottle with me when I leave the house so we have plenty of clean water to drink wherever we go. My kids use stainless steel water bottles as well, which are also an excellent choice and have the added benefit of being shatterproof. When I travel, I fill a gallon water jug made of glass and take it with us for refills.

Toxins in the Air. Toxins, Toxins, Everywhere

Before we move on to other areas of life where toxins deplete our energy, I want to point out one more type of toxin that can have major repercussions on your health. EMFs, which stands for *electromagnetic frequencies,* is the type of radiation that we are exposed to daily, mainly through our love affair with Wifi devices, such as cell phones and tablets.

Many scientists today are concerned with the effects of EMF radiation on human health, linking the use of EMF devices to increased risk of cancer, depression, and even suicide. While some argue that more research is needed before we can conclusively state that EMFs are dangerous, numerous studies have already linked them to the diseases mentioned above and more.

One way that EMFs interfere with our physiology is melatonin production. Melatonin is a hormone produced in the brain that helps regulate our circadian rhythm, also known as the "biological clock." The circadian rhythm, as we will see later, plays an integral role in our health and well-being, affecting sleep patterns, immune system regulation, and cognition. It's just one more hormone you really don't want to mess with, momma.

Unfortunately, that's exactly what EMFs do by reducing our natural levels of melatonin. While EMFs have their dangers, we all know they're not going anywhere. So, instead of trying to ban them from your life entirely, think of safer ways to use them instead. Limit the amount of time you talk on your cell phone and avoid holding it up to your ear—use headphones instead. Cell phone use has been linked to tumors in the brain and the salivary glands in the jaw, so keeping these devices away from your face as much as possible is a good idea. At home, you can turn your Wifi off or switch your devices to "airplane mode" to reduce exposure when you don't need Wi-Fi while using them. I would especially make it a point to turn off your wireless router at night while you're sleeping. This will help to reduce your overall exposure.

Phew! That's a lot of toxins we just ditched in our homes! Thankfully, limiting our exposure to toxic chemicals can be as simple as switching out our toxic products for toxin free alternatives. Keeping these chemicals out of our homes and off our skin can be one of the fastest ways to reduce the toxic load that's derailing our hormones. In the next chapter, we'll look at how to eradicate toxins in one more area you might not have even considered—your daily habits.

Chapter 7

Ditch Toxic Habits

We can't leave out the important area of daily habits in our quest to transform your health and regain your energy. Many times, fatigue stems from toxic habits that keep us from living a balanced, healthy life that's nourishing to spirit, body, and soul. Toxic habits can perpetuate the cycle of exhaustion by depleting our natural reserves of energy and the body of precious nutrients. Let's look at a few areas where toxic habits are derailing your best efforts to ditch fatigue.

Are Your Sleep Habits Toxic?

Toxic sleep habits are one of the top ways we derail our health today. It's easy to let sleep slide in our modern world, staying up late, catching our favorite sitcom or scrolling Facebook for hours when we could be happily snoozing away.

In fact, many Americans wear sleep deprivation like a badge, bragging about how little sleep they get like they deserve a medal for depriving their bodies of the daily chance to rest and repair. In our fast paced, technology-addicted society, sleep is often the first healthy habit to get booted when we need more time. That's unfortunate since the seemingly innocent act of sleep plays a major role in our overall health and (probably no surprise here) factors into our daily energy levels in a major way.

Sometimes sleep deprivation is a choice made for us, rather than a result of our own poor choices. Night shift workers, mommas caring for newborns (or toddlers who still won't sleep through the night!), and the countless people who deal with chronic insomnia, can all attest that sleep is a hot commodity for most of us. Still, our bodies don't let us off the hook just because we have a good excuse for missing our "forty winks".

There are many bodily processes that only take place when we are asleep and missing out on enough of it means our bodies—and our minds—aren't able to function optimally, creating an environment where detoxification, growth, and repair are inhibited. The liver is especially susceptible to imbalance when we are sleep deprived. We found out in chapter 4 that the liver is responsible for many of the processes of detoxification and repair in the body. When we lose out on sleep, detoxification is hindered and inflammation ramps up. Yes, my friend, that means that all those powerful detox superfoods that you've been downing are all for naught if you deprive your body of sleep on a nightly basis.

Sleep, Stress, and The Hunger Hormones

The hormones that control our appetite are also highly sensitive to the amount of sleep we log each night. Leptin, the hormone responsible for suppressing appetite, is normally created in abundance while we sleep. Ghrelin, on the other hand, is the hormone responsible for hunger and, when we deprive ourselves of much needed sleep, these two important hormones responsible for controlling the appetite become skewed.

Research has shown sleep deprivation to increase ghrelin, causing subjects to feel hungrier during the day. In fact, studies have also proved that those who shun sleep tend to be heavier than their snoozing contemporaries. The takeaway? If you're hoping to drop those extra pounds that have crept up, sleep—*not exercise*—may be your quick ticket to dropping unwanted weight.

Cortisol is another hormone that goes haywire when we don't get enough z's. When we are not getting adequate sleep, the stress hormone *cortisol* rises in response. As we've already seen, too much cortisol causes some serious issues within the body—specifically by increasing inflammation. We've also learned that inflammation is at the root of all disease, so it's not difficult to make the connection between chronic sleep deprivation and increased risk for disease, including type 2 diabetes and autoimmune disorders such as lupus, fibromyalgia, and arthritis. That's a case for logging some hours between the sheets if I've ever heard one.

Your Brain On Sleep Deprivation

Our brains don't fare any better than our other organs when we skimp on sleep either. As a matter of fact, sleep is absolutely essential for detoxification of metabolic waste produced by the brain through its normal daily functions. As your brain thinks, remembers, reasons, and uses the various hormones it uses as chemical messengers for the body, the brain produces a variety of metabolic waste products. As these metabolic wastes build up throughout the day, their accumulation is a signal to the brain that it's time for sleep. While we sleep, the body goes to work detoxifying these metabolic wastes from the brain.

Dr. Sarah Ballantyne, expert in autoimmune health and author of the definitive guide on sleep aptly named, *Go to Bed*, explains that, as we sleep, our neurons shrink by 60 percent while our flow of cerebrospinal fluid increases and specialized brain cells called *microglia* go through and sweep out the toxins that have accumulated during the day.

While I'm sure it's no surprise to find that studies have linked sleep deprivation to learning, memory, and critical thinking problems, understanding just how our brain detoxifies during sleep makes it clear how toxins in the body negatively affect both physical and mental health—and just how critical every aspect of the detoxification process is to feeling our best.

So now we know that sleep is essential to our mental and physical well-being. So, getting more sleep sounds like the obvious solution, right? Well, the short answer would be *yes*. However, there's more to a good night's sleep than just hitting the hay earlier. Let's look at some of our habits that could be setting us up for poor quality sleep so we can make sure that, when we do turn in for the night, we get the most restful, healing sleep we possibly can.

Toxic Sleep Habits

Staying Up Late

There's no way around it. Most of us need at least eight hours of sleep to function optimally. Many people require even more. When we skimp on sleep, the natural cycle of our delicate hormonal balance is skewed, creating a cascading effect on nearly every physiological process in the body. Getting less sleep than your body needs means you won't be able to fully detox, as well, since many of the important processes of detoxification only happen when you're sleeping. Do yourself a favor and don't skimp on sleep.

Sleeping with Electronics

As modern and technologically-advanced as society has become, there's just no fooling Mother Nature. While modern conveniences, like smartphones and iPads, certainly make life easier and more fun, they have their downside as well. And, if you're sleeping with your electronic devices close at hand, you're getting an unhealthy dose of those toxic side effects all night long.

Electronic devices, especially those that emit a Wifi signal, create electromagnetic disturbances that interfere with our sensitive circadian rhythms, disrupting our sleep/wake cycles, and making it difficult to get a good night's sleep.

While I was going through my health coaching program, I remember our instructor recounting a situation with one of her clients that really brought home the point of just how toxic EMFs can be to a good night's sleep. During one of her group coaching sessions, a client, who was having trouble staying asleep at night, asked for some tips on how she could finally end the cycle of waking up throughout the night, often unable to fall back asleep for several hours. One of the instructor's main suggestions was to remove the electronic devices from the client's bedroom while she was sleeping at night. Amazingly, the client reported back the next week that the only change she made to her lifestyle was to nix electronics in the bedroom and her sleeping troubles completely disappeared.

Keeping the Lights On

As if EMFs weren't enough of a reason to keep the electronics out of the bedroom, here's one more: Blue light emitted by electronic devices and overhead lights also disrupt our circadian rhythms. Blue light is the same type of light we get from the sun and it signals the body that it's daytime and we should be awake. That's a good thing during the day when we spend time outdoors soaking up the sun's rays. The body gets the message to stay awake and energetic during the day and regulates the hormones that control our sleep/wake cycles so we can sleep restfully at night.

When we're bombarded by blue light at the wrong time from electronic devices, it sends confusing signals to the brain about when we should be awake and when we should be sleeping. You'll have a harder time winding down at night if you spend a lot of time in front of the TV or iPad before going to bed. You're not Motel 6, so do yourself a favor and *leave the lights off*!

Set Yourself Up For a Great Night's Sleep

If so many of the habits we've cultivated as a society around sleep are leaving us exhausted and irritable all day long, what's the solution to a great night's sleep? Let's break down the components to your best z's.

Go To Bed Early

If staying up late is killing your mojo, the obvious solution is to go to bed earlier. But, how do you know how much sleep you really need? The best way to find out is to experiment with your bedtime. To get a good eight hours of uninterrupted sleep, decide what time you want to wake up in the morning and then count backwards eight hours. Then, add an extra half hour to allow yourself time to really get comfortable and relaxed before sleep kicks in.

Give your new bedtime a try for a few days and note how you feel. Still feeling tired and run down throughout the day? Move your bedtime up by half an hour until you find the perfect window of sleep time that leaves you feeling your best. Then, be sure to guard your bedtime like a dog with a bone. Make it a priority for the sake of your health to get to bed on time every night as much as possible.

Create a Cozy Sleeping Environment

We already know that EMFs from electronics and artificial light can disrupt our natural sleep cycle. Once you've removed the electronic devices from the bedroom (or, if that's not possible, at least move them as far away from you as you can), be sure to make the room as dark as possible during sleeping hours. Blackout curtains can help immensely if you live in a brightly lit area. Even a small amount of light can interfere with good sleep, so be diligent to block out as much light as you can.

I've been experimenting with this one myself and can attest that, by keeping the room very dark by covering my alarm clock, using room-darkening curtains, and keeping the door shut to nix hallway light has made a big difference in the quality of my sleep. Which has made a big difference in the quality of my energy levels during the day. Honestly, I wish I had taken my own advice earlier and kept the room dark while trying to sleep.

Other factors that can make or break your nightly siesta include the temperature of your room and the noise level. A dip in temperature at bedtime signals the body to relax and sleep restfully, and taking a warm bath is a great way to send that signal. The rise in body temperature from the warm bath, followed by the subsequent dip in temperature when you get out send the signal to the brain that you're ready for sleep.

Ideally, the temperature of your bedroom should be on the cool side, around 70 degrees F. Using a fan can help to keep you cool while sleeping and provide a bit of white noise to drown out any sounds that might keep you awake. The cooler temps will help your body recognize that it's time to sleep.

Get Some Natural Light

While artificial light in the evening has a detrimental effect on our ability to fall and stay asleep, the truth is we do need light—it just needs to be the right kind and at the right time. The *circadian rhythm* refers to the cycle of physiological processes our bodies go through in a 24-hour period and the amount of natural sunlight we are exposed to daily has a huge modulating effect on this cycle. In human speak, that simply means our bodies use light from the sun to set the cycle of rest and wakefulness we need to be truly productive throughout the day and to sleep soundly each night.

The process of setting our circadian rhythm is controlled by the circadian clock, a part of the brain responsible for controlling the hormones that regulate the sleep-wake cycle. When our skin is exposed to natural light, hormones are released that signal the body it's time to be awake. Miss out on your daily dose of sunlight and your sleep hormones can run the risk of getting skewed.

Do You Deal With Stress In a Toxic Way?

I hear so many women talking about the struggle these days. You know—*The Struggle*. The frustration of trying to raise kids who are morally upright, polite in public, and actually dressed in matching clothes. Of getting dinner on the table, the dog fed, the laundry done, and (is it possible?) put away. Not to mention keeping your hubby happy ;), organizing the school bake sale, and running the church women's ministry (or just remembering to bring the snacks to the next meeting). The list goes on and on. Feeling guilty because we can't be everything to everyone, we add more and more to our plates while ignoring the internal signals to stop and nourish *yourself*—spirit, soul, and body.

It's almost a badge of honor these days to push ourselves past our natural limits and be supermom. From supermodels staring back at us on the cover of fashion magazines in the grocery line to the gorgeous mom in our playgroup who looks like she has it all together, we're constantly bombarded with messages of how we don't measure up.

While I can't personally go through the magazines in your grocery store's checkout aisle and hide the fashion magazines behind a copy of *National Geographic* (hopefully you look better than a 3,000-year-old mummy), what I can do is encourage you to find a better way to look at your life and deal with the stress that's always waiting to bring you to your proverbial knees.

Stop and take a moment to think about the way you deal with stress in your life. Do you binge on Ben & Jerry's after the kids go to bed? "Check out" with your favorite Netflix show before turning in? Complain to a girlfriend on the phone for a few hours? While all of these ways of coping with stress may make you feel temporary relief, the problem is just that—they're temporary. There's nothing wrong with any of these activities—except when they become a crutch to cope with the stress of life. They may make you feel better in the moment, but they haven't really helped you make progress towards truly managing the stress in your life.

What if you built some routines (habits!) into your day that not only helped you relax and feel better, but moved you towards your ultimate goals of being the best mom and wife you can be? After all, the dairy and sugar high you get from eating ice cream probably doesn't serve your ultimate goal of nourishing your gut and ditching the toxic foods that are draining you of energy, right? ;) Instead, let's develop some healthy ways of relieving stress that not only feel great in the moment, but will have you feeling amazing long after. Personally, I love carving small, quiet moments into my day that put me in tune with my desires, as well as choosing some more focused and intentional ways to de-stress. Here are a few of my favorites:

Detox Baths

A fun way to ditch stress, while simultaneously ramping up your detox pathways, is to take a relaxing detox bath. Detox baths consist of adding some fun ingredients to a warm bath and soaking for at least 20 minutes.

While there are many things you can throw into the tub to create a lovely detox bath, I suggest starting with Epsom salts and maybe a few drops of a relaxing essential oil, such as lavender. The Epsom salts are a great source of magnesium, a mineral that promotes relaxation in the body and can help you sleep better. This makes detox baths a great way to unwind before bed. A cup of baking soda can also be beneficial in moving out toxins during a bath, as can raw apple cider vinegar and sea salts. Simply take a cup of any one of these ingredients and add it to a very warm bath. Ideally, the water will be hot, but not uncomfortable. This helps to draw the toxins out as you relax.

Dry Brushing

Dry brushing is another way to get a pretty momma-glow while helping to stimulate the flow of *lymph* (detox!). If you've never tried it, you can check out my article on how to dry brush here: www.overcomingauto.com/dry-skin-brushing/. Essentially, you take a brush made specifically for this purpose and brush your skin, starting at your feet and working your way up, using long strokes on your limbs and a circular motion on your abdomen and back. This action not only helps encourage the flow of lymph through the body, it also exfoliates the skin, removing dead skin cells and toxins that have been released through the skin.

Start slowly when you begin dry brushing, with light strokes until you can work up to firmer strokes. I also recommend only dry brushing once or twice a week so that you don't strip your skin of the delicate oils that are responsible for keeping your skin hydrated and protected.

Journaling

Journaling is yet another way I love to de-stress. This is a popular habit with many people and can really help you tune into what's going on in your life to ramp up your stress levels in the first place. Journaling also provides a great opportunity to really check in with yourself on what's working (or not working) for you in your life right now. Take the opportunity to think back over your day and take note of your moods, shifts in your energy level, and what foods you consumed that day. You may just catch a pattern in how a certain food affects your energy or thinking you wouldn't otherwise have noticed if you weren't tuning in to the situation through journaling.

Do Your Thing

While there are countless ways to reduce stress in a healthy way, the key takeaway here is to find a way that works for you. I love taking walks outside in nature. Perhaps, for you, it's dancing or sewing or reading. A friend of mine recently discovered that she loves Jazzercise, not only for the physical exercise, but for the boost of feel-good endorphins she gets as well. Whatever method you choose to de-stress, just make sure it's something you will feel just as good about the next day as you do in the moment. I think that *might* cross Ben & Jerry's off the list. *Just sayin'*.

Toxic Eating Habits

Before we move on to our last area of toxins, I want to do a check-in on a few other toxic habits that may seem small but can have a huge impact on your health. While we spent a whole chapter on what you should and shouldn't eat to keep your system free of toxins and full of nutrients, we didn't address *how* you eat. And how you eat can make a big difference in your body's ability to digest and assimilate the nutrients in your meal.

Relax! (and Eat!)

The first toxic habit many of us have surrounding our eating habits involves the environment we're eating in—both the physical and mental environment. If you're like most people in our fast-paced society, you probably do a lot of eating on the run, rushing through your lunch break or even (heaven forbid) working through lunch, gulping down food while managing your "to do" list. It's not uncommon to see many people with a Wifi device in front of their faces while eating (guilty-as-charged here).

If you're not taking the time to relax and enjoy your meals, your digestion suffers. Whenever possible, choose a comfortable environment to eat in, preferably with pleasant people you enjoy being with (easier said than done, I know). Nix eating in front of the TV or doing other things while eating, such as reading or checking your email. Instead, take time to not just eat, but *enjoy* your meal. Look at your food—notice the appetizing colors, textures, and smells. Have you ever noticed how just thinking about your favorite meal can have you salivating? The process of digestion starts in the brain—before you even take your first bite.

As your mind anticipates enjoying your meal, you begin to produce enzymes and hormones that stimulate digestion. What I'm getting at here is this: By taking the time to relax and enjoy your meal, the process of digestion is vastly improved. Stress, such as eating in a rushed environment, and dividing our attention between too many things, slows down the digestive process by arousing the parasympathetic nervous system, which means the proper signals to begin the digestive process get ignored.

You've probably experienced this if you've tried to eat while you were really stressed out. Did you notice it gave you a stomach ache, heartburn, or other unpleasant symptoms? Stressful eating habits, including eating too quickly, can derail your best efforts at healthy digestion. Many people suffer from digestive discomfort simply because they don't take the time to properly chew their food, gulping it down mindlessly. Remember to chew each bite thoroughly before swallowing, putting your fork down between bites, and really being present with your meal and the company you are in. Your digestive system will thank you.

Healthy Moving

There's one habit we need to look at that can make or break your energy levels. Healthy moving habits play an important role in regulating our hormones and boosting the immune system. Thankfully, it doesn't take hours in the gym to reap the benefits of healthy movement. At the same time, many of us aren't getting enough healthy movement each day.

Healthy moving goes beyond what you probably think of when you hear the word *exercise*. We humans were meant to be mobile—walking, reaching, lifting, and moving around throughout the day. All this activity helps to stimulate lymph flow, improve digestion, and strengthen muscles and bones. Because of our modern lifestyle habit of sitting way too much, we are often lacking in the movement nutrients we need to stay healthy.

While setting aside time to exercise each day is important, it's equally important to remember to move *throughout* the day. A thirty-minute jaunt on the treadmill simply can't undo the negative effects of sitting for eight hours a day at a desk. To combat the negative effects of being too sedentary, start to develop a practice of moving throughout the day.

Set a timer for twenty minutes and, when it goes off, get up from your computer and stretch for a few minutes before going back to work. Try alternating your positions during the day as well. If you usually sit at a desk to work, try elevating your computer and standing for part of your day or even sitting on the floor where you can stretch your legs out for a few minutes. These small changes in the way you move throughout the day can have a big impact on your overall health.

For more information on how to weave healthy moving into your day without feeling like you have to spend a lot of time or effort exercising, check out the website *HealthyMoving.com*. The classes offered on this site have completely revolutionized the way I think of movement and exercise and taught me how to effortlessly make healthy moving a part of my day.

Habits Will Move You Forward

Getting your habits under control in the way you sleep, the way you eat, and the way you move will help you make major strides toward recovering your energy and regulating your hormones. Choose one of the habits we discussed in this chapter and start working towards making it a *daily* habit. Then, once you've mastered getting to bed on time, for example, move on to changing your eating habits by paying close attention to your eating environment. Trying to change too many habits at once can feel overwhelming and usually results in giving up before the new habits are firmly entrenched in your thinking.

Remember, a habit is something you do at the same time and in the same place to the point that you don't even have to think about it or remind yourself to do it. While some of these changes may seem difficult at first, if you keep at them day after day, soon they'll be routine. Next, we'll look at another area where ditching the toxins can have a major impact on your energy and hormones. Even how you can use the power of habit in this critical area to transform your health—the area of *your thoughts*.

Chapter 8
Ditch Toxic Thoughts

When I think of all the toxins we are being attacked with on a daily basis from all the sources we've already discussed, *frustrating* is the word that comes to mind. Yet, with all the toxins that threaten us from the outside, some of the most destructive toxins are those that come from within in the form of our own thoughts.

You may be familiar with this statistic: *Over 90 percent of disease is stress-related.* We've all heard it before and nod our heads knowingly, thinking it only applies to overweight businessmen battling the high stress corporate world. Unfortunately, no one is immune to the effects of stress. In fact, stress isn't so much a product of our environment as it is a product of how we *perceive* our environment. The way we think about and interpret the situations we find ourselves in daily directly influences our health.

Just because the environment you find yourself in isn't one that people typically associate with a high stress lifestyle, doesn't mean that it's not stressful *for you*. The mom who feels overwhelmed at the thought of putting healthy meals on the table, getting laundry done, and making time for her hubby each night is just as prone to stress-related illness as the CEO of the Fortune 500 company whose decisions influence thousands of people and involve millions of dollars.

You might remember from my story in the beginning of this book that ditching the toxins in my diet made a huge impact on my health. I suddenly found myself with more energy, mental clarity, and enthusiasm than I had felt in *years*. **I felt like a different person.** Can I let you in on a little secret, though? While I did experience quite a bit of relief from my health problems by committing to a healthier diet, my transformation was a long road that took several years of ups and downs. I found that my diet wasn't the only area toxins were attacking. Toxic thoughts were leaving me drained and depressed. It wasn't until I committed to taking control over my thoughts that I saw real strides in my healing journey. While taking back your mental real estate may not be the easiest step in your journey towards glowing health, I promise it will be worth the fight.

The Science of Thought

For many people, it can seem a little mystical to assert that thoughts can have a direct physical impact on our health. After all, we understand how eating cookies can cause the scale to tip unfavorably—too many calories consumed equates to the excess being stored as fat, right? It's simple science—calories in, calories out—kinda thing that we can easily grasp. So, how can our thoughts, something so intangible and fleeting, directly impact physical matter in a way that shapes our bodies for better or worse?

Science is finally providing answers to these questions—and those answers are truly astounding. Scientists once thought of the brain as a sort of machine—input in, input out—that was hardwired during our early years. Something that was fixed and unchangeable as we aged and the inevitable decline of physical and mental health set in. However, new research in the field of neuroscience has changed the way we view the mind and what it is capable of. For one, scientists now know that the brain is, in fact, able to change, to rewire itself and even regenerate after damage. Scientists call this ability of the brain to change and adapt in response to the environment *neuroplasticity*— and it's the reason why, no matter how poor your thinking may be now, you do have the ability to change it for the better.

Allow me to share a powerful example of how your thinking can shape your life. If you're a fan of TED Talks, you've probably seen social psychologist Amy Cuddy's twenty minute presentation on *presence*—our non-verbal cues that communicate to others and ourselves how we wish to be treated. (If you haven't seen it, check it out on *YouTube*—it's totally worth the watch!) While Cuddy, a researcher at Harvard, focuses her talk on body language and how it affects your outlook and attitude, something amazing happens during the brief but powerful time she takes the stage.

As Cuddy later shares in her book, aptly named *Presence*, her talk took an unexpectedly personal turn when she decided to take a chance on sharing her own trial with overcoming severe mental health issues after an auto accident left her struggling to function normally. After being thrown from the vehicle, Cuddy woke up to find herself in a head injury rehab ward where she was told that she had little hope of finishing college.

As someone for whom school had always come easily, this was bad news indeed. But Cuddy completed college nonetheless, finally graduating four years later than planned. Even more amazing, Cuddy went on to continue her education at Princeton. However, her disabilities had left her doubting her chances of completing the rigors of graduate school.

Fortunately for Cuddy, she had an advisor who wouldn't let her quit. On the verge of dropping out right before one particularly challenging speech she was scheduled to give, her advisor pushed her to stay and, essentially, to "fake it 'til you make it"—and not just until you make it, but *until you become it*. Cuddy went on to not only finish graduate school, but become one of the top social psychology researchers in the country. She accomplished the very thing she was told was impossible for her to do. That's the power of believing in your own abilities to overcome any obstacle.

This story, and the countless other amazing stories of struggle and triumph just like it, bear out the fact that our brains are remarkably adept at changing and regenerating through the power of thought and belief. When Jesus said, "All things are possible to him who believes," he was stating what science is just now beginning to prove out. Your thoughts and beliefs shape your life—for better or for worse. How exactly *do* our thoughts change the physical DNA of our brains—and the rest of the body for that matter?

Thinking Influences Genes

Understanding how thoughts affect genetic expression shows us that we truly can change our health with our thoughts. According to Dr. Caroline Leaf, author of *Switch On Your Brain*, our thoughts turn sets of genes on and off in complex relationships. In *Switch On Your Brain,* Dr. Leaf explains that, "Molecules are assembled into proteins by the genetic instructions in our DNA. These instructions dictate the anatomy and physiology of our bodies, and **we control up to 90 percent of this process through our thinking**."

In fact, research has been able to show how DNA changes in response to our thoughts. One study conducted by the Institute of HeartMath demonstrated that emotions, such as fear and anger, caused DNA to change shape—coiling up and become shorter—which inhibited genetic expression. Positive feelings, such as love, gratitude, and appreciation, however, reversed this shortening of DNA so that genetic expression was uninhibited.

The study also looked at HIV-positive patients and found that positive thoughts and emotions increased their resistance to disease 300,000 times more than those who lacked these positive feelings. While there is still much research to be done on exactly how thoughts influence genes, the takeaway here is that your thoughts, feelings, and emotions affect your genes and, thus, the health of your body.

Fascinating stuff, isn't it? Your thoughts are powerful, friend. And while that may be an exciting realization, it's not always easy to change those thought patterns that have been deeply ingrained in our minds over a lifetime. They can change, however, as we've just seen. Ditching toxic thoughts requires you to first identify the thoughts that are keeping you stuck and then replace them with thoughts that are healing and empowering.

While many experts emphasize either the biological component of mental health or the psychological/spiritual component, the truth is, both pieces come into play when it comes to staying mentally strong. Without the nutrients necessary to produce neurotransmitters, our brain simply won't function properly. Yet, you still have the responsibility to choose the right thoughts and deny access to toxic thoughts. Easier said than done, I know.

Types of Toxic Thinking

Defining what constitutes toxic thinking isn't exactly brain surgery (ha, ha). However, I want to highlight a few types of thinking that are especially toxic and interfere with the body's innate healing abilities. Start paying attention to the types of thoughts that are drifting in and out of your mind during the day, especially your self-talk. What you're telling yourself *about yourself* is having a powerful effect on your life and your health. Are your thoughts about yourself uplifting and healing? Or, do some of the types of toxic thoughts below mark your thinking?

Guilt and Shame

Dr. Brené Brown, author of *Daring Greatly,* could easily be called *the* expert on the topic of shame. According to Dr. Brown, "Shame is the intensely painful feeling that we are unworthy of love and belonging. It's the idea that we are fundamentally flawed and, therefore, unworthy of connection." Sounds like pretty intense stuff, doesn't it? Yet, no one is immune to the damaging effects of shame. We've all know that feeling of being flawed and the secret fear that deep down we're unlovable. In fact, Dr. Brown declares emphatically that shame is lethal—as we carry guilt and shame around, stewing in it for years. It begins to affect our actions, color our responses to others, and, yes, even impact our health.

Fear and Anxiety

Fear is another soul sucking emotion that depletes our strength. Like shame and guilt, fear is paralyzing. As a matter of fact, that's the main problem with negative emotions in general. When we feel ashamed—and therefore, unworthy—we stop ourselves from seeking the love and grace that can set us free, thinking we don't deserve it. When we're fearful, we hold back from making the very decisions that can push us past our own resistance. In other words, we *stay stuck*.

Fear involves focusing on negative thoughts and outcomes rather than focusing on what's possible. Fear robs you of the joy of the moment because of your focus on "what could be" in the future. Meanwhile, you miss out on the beauty of this moment—and your health most definitely suffers.

Unforgiveness and Blame

Playing the "blame game" is a sure-fire way to stay stuck in the same sad story as well. When we refuse to forgive others of their wrongs— even blaming them for our circumstances—we cripple ourselves from moving forward. While the other negative emotions we've looked at have been inwardly focused, unforgiveness and blame place the focus squarely on the shoulders of another. While it may take some of the pressure off yourself to blame others, it also means that you are giving the power to control your life to someone else.

The truth is, no matter what has happened to you, or what other people have done to you, you can rise above it and overcome it. And, if that's true, then the only person who's really keeping you from living the fulfilling life you desire is *yourself*. Holding on to blame and unforgiveness puts us squarely in the seat of a victim—a place where our life is outside of our control and others hold the power over our lives. It's time to give these negative emotions the boot!

Overcoming Negative Emotions

So, how does one overcome all the negative voices in your head and focus on healing, positive thinking that will move your life forward? Moving forward, after all, is what life's all about. You weren't meant to stay stuck in the same place year after miserable year, wishing things were different but feeling powerless to change your circumstances. It's great to know that positive thinking can change DNA and alter brain chemistry in a positive way. But to be honest, that probably doesn't do much to motivate you to move forward.

Getting out of the negative emotions and changing your thinking can be tough. As damaging as we know those negative emotions to be, the truth is, we are getting something out of them. By blaming others, we don't have to take the responsibility for our own mistakes. Fear keeps us in our comfort zone, protecting us from the unknown instead of stepping out into what could be (and, after all, what if what *could be* is something bad?)

I have experienced first-hand what it's like to be stuck in a never-ending cycle of negative emotions that feel safe and comfortable, yet disempowering and depressing at the same time. Looking back, I never really recognized how much negative emotions controlled me. Really, I suffered from depression, often crying over things that had happened years ago and, sometimes, even things that hadn't happened at all!

For instance, I used to pull up my bank account online to record transactions in my checkbook register and be furious if I saw that my husband had spent $20! Money was tight at the time and he had a bad habit of spending money without recording the amount. But, in the grand scheme of things, my reaction was over the top. This would usually happen while I was getting ready to leave work for the day and I would fume all the way to my car and back home at his irresponsibility, imagining what else he was probably doing that he had never told me about. Often, I would cry all the way to daycare to pick up my kids, trying to pull myself together so my daycare provider didn't think I was a total nut job. Honestly, it all sounds crazy now but, back then, I didn't really recognize that I had a problem. It was such an ingrained pattern that I didn't even realize how unhealthy my thoughts and behavior were.

It took a lot of time to change my thought patterns. First, I had to own up to the fact that my thoughts were self-destructive—not something any of us like to admit. Then, I had to start replacing those negative thinking patterns with new thoughts that put me squarely in control of my own life and future. To be honest, it was a scary place to be sometimes. Yet, I'm glad I finally decided to nix those negative thought patterns and start making better decisions. I'm convinced I would still be stuck in the same sad place of depression and anxiety if I hadn't taken the steps I needed to ditch toxic thinking.

I wish I could give you a neat little list of positive ways to cope with your emotions and you could simply fill out a checklist each day to keep yourself on track. Oh, if only it were that easy. Let's face it, just like in my story, negative emotions can become a learned pattern—something we may not even recognize we're doing. Sounds a lot like a habit, doesn't it? Well, that's good and bad news. The bad news is that habits can be hard to change. The good news is that habits *can* be changed. Yeah, I know the good and bad news sound pretty much the same, but that's because they pretty much are. While a bad habit can be hard to break, once a positive habit is set in place it can be equally hard to break. Which is exactly what we want.

Habits are a favorite topic of mine because, when I learned that I could radically change my life just by changing some of the small, seemingly insignificant actions that were part of my daily routine, I felt like I had hit the jackpot. It meant I didn't have to be a victim to my thoughts, my emotions, or even my choices. I could change all of them by changing my habits. Since we delved into habit formation in the last chapter, I'm not going to reinvent the wheel here. Suffice it to say that the same way you create habits in any area of life—sleep habits, exercise habits, or what have you—is the same way you change your habits around toxic thinking.

Let me sum it up in three words just to make it super simple: *You keep practicing*. You find a new way of dealing with your thoughts and you start training yourself to replace old habits with new techniques. You do it over and over. And when you mess up and find yourself slipping back into old habits, you pick yourself up, dust yourself off, and go again. It's really that simple. Ok, *simple* probably isn't the best word because you'll be tempted to get frustrated and discouraged and even give up. But (and this is a big *but*!) if you just keep at it—it will work!

If you're ready to replace some old, negative toxic thinking with a new outlook, then let's dive into a few of the top ways to step into your place of healing and wholeness. I want to share with you the types of thoughts that should mark your thinking if you want to start transforming your health—as well as some ways to build healthy thought habits into your daily routine that will put your life in forward motion fast.

Train Yourself to Focus On Positive Thoughts

The key to ditching toxic thinking isn't just to stop thinking negative thoughts. To be successful, you'll have to replace negative thinking with something else. Instead of guilt, shame, fear, and unforgiveness, you can begin, moment by moment, to choose thoughts of faith, of grace, and of forgiveness—both for yourself and others.

Faith

As Dr. Leaf writes in *Switch On Your Brain*, we as humans are programmed for faith. "We are wired for love, which means our mental circuitry is wired only for the positive, and we have a natural optimism bias wired into us." Sounds like we were created for faith, if you ask me.

I've heard all kinds of definitions for faith, but one of my favorites is this: *Faith is simply our response to God's grace*. Faith is powerful, but don't over complicate it. Faith is really a simple act of trust on your part in response to God's goodness. Faith is believing that good things are in store for you and that there is an answer to every challenge you're facing because there is a God who loves you and has good things planned for your life—things like good health and a strong mind.

Faith is so vital to your success in overcoming health issues, like exhaustion and depression, because, if you don't believe, *truly believe*, that you can get well—that you are, in fact, *supposed* to get well—your chances of success are greatly diminished. However, when you find in the Word that God promises to restore your health and heal your wounds (Jeremiah 30), then you can respond to that promise by choosing to believe that things can and will get better.

Grace

We've already mentioned grace, but what exactly is it? Like faith, it may seem to be some mystical, spiritual concept that no one really understands but you know you're supposed to nod your head wisely whenever it's mentioned. Grasping the concept of grace, however, is vital to using your faith. I've heard grace defined as God's unmerited favor and I love that definition. It's God's love and acceptance of us despite what we have or haven't done to earn it.

Grace is an easy concept for me to grasp when I look at my own children. Sometimes they make mistakes, do things to frustrate and disappoint me—yet none of that changes my love and acceptance for them one iota. I accept them simply because they're mine. They belong to me and, no matter what happens between us, nothing could possibly change that love.

Can you relate to loving someone that way? Then why do we think God would feel any differently about us, his very own creation? Grace is the opposite of shame. Where shame makes you feel unworthy and unacceptable, grace says, "You are worthy. You are accepted. Simply because you are mine." Talk about a freeing thought! When you grasp the concept of grace, you grasp the concept of your own self-worth. You can finally understand your worthiness to be loved, to be well, and to be happy and successful. Grace is one of the most powerful concepts in this universe and it's yours for the taking.

Forgiveness

When someone hurts us, it's painful and we feel totally justified in our response to blame them. Forgiveness is often the last thing we want to give to the one who caused us pain. It may help to realize that forgiveness isn't really about the person who hurt you. It's about yourself. When you release the person who hurt you from their debt against you, you're really releasing yourself from the cage of unforgiveness so you can move on to bigger and better things.

That's not to say forgiveness is easy. It's not about stuffing down the emotions of hurt or anger you feel towards the wrongdoer. It's about experiencing those emotions, accepting that you were hurt, and then choosing to move past the pain for your own sake. While you may experience pain from what others have done, you can choose, on purpose, to move past the negative feelings of blame and unforgiveness. Why waste mental real estate on blame and unforgiveness? You're destined for an amazing life of health and wholeness, so don't sabotage that plan with toxic thoughts like unforgiveness. Do yourself a favor and let it go, friend. You'll be so glad you did.

Ditch Toxic Mental Habits

Ok, we've tackled some of the bigger issues of changing toxic thinking. Before we leave this subject for other pastures, however, I want to focus in on the more practical side of ditching toxic thoughts. After all, it's usually not enough to know you *should* do something if you don't know *how* to do it. Knowing you should eat better is a whole lot different than having the practical tools in place to carry it out, no? After all, "eat better" for some people means choosing a low-fat granola bar over a Snickers—and we've already seen that's not much of an improvement. The same concept applies to our thoughts. It's one thing to know we should think positive thoughts—but what does that look like on a day-to-day basis? Let's look at a few of my favorite mental habits that will keep your thoughts strong and healthy.

The Drain of Technology

It's said that the average American watches six hours of television a day. Six hours! Considering that the vast majority of content on the TV could be most definitely classified in the negative category, it's no wonder toxic thinking is such a problem for many people. Social media is just as pervasive, and often just as pessimistic as television. Yet, many people spend all day with their smartphone in front of their faces, checking their Facebook status and posting selfies to Instagram.

Obviously, you know where I'm going with this one. If you want to turn your thoughts in a more uplifting direction, the first step is to stop feeding your mind with the mental junk food that technology provides in the form of sitcoms and social media. Again, easier said than done, but, as with so many of the choices that make our lives healthier and happier, the effort of self-discipline is worth the reward of a peaceful mind and energetic body.

Turn It Off!

The best way to dial down the technology habit is to simply turn it off. Make it a habit to shut off the television after you've watched your favorite show instead of leaving the tube turned on to whatever happens to pop up next. Same with social media. Turn notifications on your smartphone off so you don't find yourself checking your phone 14,000 times a day, responding to each ding like one of Pavlov's dogs salivating for a treat at the sound of a bell. Shut down the computer when you've finished checking your email.

Set aside a specific time each day to check in on social media and then leave it alone. I check my email first thing in the morning and then again in the afternoon—and I make myself leave it be until it's time. You'll be surprised at how much time you're really wasting doing things like checking social media and email because you "don't want to miss something important." By setting aside a specific time to indulge in technology, you'll find yourself not only missing out on much of the depressing drivel, you'll also be more efficient with your time.

Reign In Your Obligations

Speaking of technology, it's amazing how it has opened a world of possibilities to all of us in so many arenas. It's possible to travel the globe (both literally and virtually), connect with people around the world, learn almost anything via the online world, and get just about any answer we need by googling it. We live in truly amazing times, but there is a downside to our fast-paced society that many people don't recognize—too many obligations. We live in the "do it all, have it all" age and, for most women, the pressure to be supermom is seldom far from our minds.

One of the reasons many women are struggling with keeping their health in line is that they are simply pulled in too many directions. This lack of focus does what? First of all, it can create feelings of overwhelm which only serve to drain our mental energy further. Secondly, it means you're most likely not spending the time needed on your true priorities—if you even know what those are.

The quick fix here? Sit down with pen and paper and list out your top priorities, such as your family and marriage, your health, your career, finances, etc. Under each category, decide what actions you need to take to make those priorities happen and then use that list to decide which activities in your life are moving you towards your goals and which are just distracting you from your true priorities and need to be nixed.

If driving your kids to endless activities is draining your energy, negating your ability to get healthy meals on the table, and depleting your family of truly meaningful interactions, maybe it's time to ditch a few of those extracurricular activities. Let the kids pick one activity and let the others go. Your marriage, your waistline, and, yes, even your kids, just might thank you.

Develop a Mindset Practice

One of my top ways to reign in toxic thinking is through a mindset practice. Simply put, a mindset practice involves setting aside some time to specifically focus in on the mental and spiritual habits that will bring about the positive results you're aiming for. I love to spend the first part of my day focusing my thoughts and energy towards what I truly want to achieve. In fact, creating a mindset practice has been one of the most instrumental habits I've developed to move my life and my health forward.

My mindset practice involves spending time with God, both through prayer and reading the Word, as well as reviewing my goals, speaking out positive affirmations over my life, and reading from an uplifting book. Your mindset practice can be whatever inspires you and helps you focus in on the thoughts that keep you moving forward. Try journaling, reading a devotional, or exercising to help get yourself into a positive mental mindset. In my book, *Make Your Day*, I share five of the top morning habits practiced by the world's most successful people. If you need some help getting your morning mindset routine started, I'd recommend checking it out.

Spend Time With the Right People

If you're still struggling to keep toxic thinking at bay, look at the people you spend time with. While you may not be able to do anything about the snarky gossipmongers in your office who keep up a constant stream of negativity, you can choose whether or not you participate. I've noticed that there are a few people in my life who tend to have something negative to say whenever I'm around them. I also noticed that, when I spend time with them, I tend towards negativity as well. Deciding to minimize the amount of time I spend with those people helped me focus on keeping my thoughts positive.

On the other hand, there are a few people in my life who always seem to inspire and encourage me. Do you have that one friend who you know will always be happy to celebrate your accomplishments and share your joy? Is there a certain family member who challenges you to go for more in life and stop playing small? Positive people will leave their mark on your life just as surely as the negative people. Take some time to think about who you spend time with and make it a point to choose your friends carefully.

Practice Gratitude

I love the way Terri Savelle Foy describes the power of gratitude in her book, *Imagine Big*: "Your mind is like a magnet—whatever gets in your mind and stays there, you will attract in your life. When you practice gratitude for what you have and for what you are expecting, you literally attract more to be grateful for."

Many high achievers have made gratitude a daily practice in their lives. Take a cue from those who use the power of gratitude and list out the things you are grateful for on a daily basis. Grab a journal and make a list of three things (or more) you are thankful for—from your kids to your favorite pair of undies— nothing is too big or too small to appreciate.

By the way, gratitude is your highest expression of faith. When you thank God, not only for what he has done, but for what you believe he is doing, you are showing him that you believe him despite the circumstances. In the book of Acts, Paul and Silas found themselves stuck in prison. Cold, hungry, and bleeding from the nasty beating they had received, they began to loudly praise God. How do we know it was loud? The scripture tells us that the other prisoners heard them! This was no half-hearted praise of empty words. Guess what happened next? The doors swung open and Paul and Silas walked right out of those prison doors.

When you express praise and thanksgiving, doors of opportunity will open for you too. If you're ready to make gratitude more than just a feel-good ritual you practice at the dinner table, and are interested in harnessing the power of thanksgiving to truly catapult your faith forward, don't forget to practice this powerful mental habit daily.

Read For Healthy Thoughts

This is one of the fastest ways to develop a healing mindset and change your thinking. Spending time focusing on the right thoughts and ideas can completely transform your thinking, and books that help you cultivate the right type of thinking are priceless. Reading can challenge your thinking and offer new solutions to help move your life forward. I make it a point to read at least one book each month that helps me develop a growth mindset—one of the most notable characteristics of highly successful people.

When To Get Help

Sometimes, despite our best efforts to change our thinking, we're plagued with toxic thoughts that seem to overpower our best intentions to move forward in life. When your thoughts seem to be controlling you—instead of the other way around—it can be frightening and demoralizing. The best thing you can do is reach out to someone who can help to safely guide you through the rough waters of overcoming toxic thinking.

If you feel overwhelmed by fear, anxiety, or depression, it's important to talk to someone in your life who can help you get things back on track. A trusted friend, pastor, or professional counselor can make a huge difference in helping you regain your perspective and ditch the toxic thinking. If you feel that you need the extra help, I encourage you to find someone who can give you the support you need while you work on transforming your thoughts.

Your thoughts are just as powerful in transforming your health as the foods you eat or the amount of exercise you log daily. Don't make the mistake I did for many years and try to overcome poor health simply by eating better, getting more sleep, or taking the right supplements. Your life will rise to the level of your thoughts, so start developing healthy thought patterns now and your mind and body will thank you for years to come.

Let's look at one last area where toxins can disrupt our best efforts to regain our energy and reset our hormones. You may be surprised to learn that underlying infections in the gut and elsewhere in the body can be disrupting your health and depleting your energy levels. In the next chapter, we'll look at some of the most common infections that can be responsible for fatigue, thyroid disease, and autoimmunity—and how you can identify and eradicate them fast so you can start feeling amazing.

Chapter 9
Ditch Toxic Infections

When stubborn health issues don't seem to respond to diet and lifestyle changes, it's time to consider if darker forces are at work. Specifically, I'm talking about underlying infections which can create toxic by-products that interrupt normal cell function and incite the cycle of inflammation and illness. As toxins in the body begin to accumulate, changes in body chemistry can create an internal environment that encourages the growth of pathogenic bacteria, fungus, and parasites.

These infections can be difficult to pinpoint because they can do their dirty work within the body for years, with symptoms that are often nonspecific—or even presenting with no symptoms at all. Many people live with these latent infections for years without realizing it, until other annoying health issues begin to crop up, such as autoimmune disease or even just the vague and frustrating symptoms of exhaustion, brain fog, and digestive issues that most of us shrug off as the inevitable signs of aging.

I learned firsthand how underlying infections can derail your best efforts to ditch fatigue and live a healthy life back when I began my journey into ditching the toxic foods and chemicals that were at the root of my autoimmune thyroid health problems. After removing some of the most toxic foods from my diet—gluten, dairy, and soy products—I noticed that my health did improve, somewhat. The joint pain I experienced began to fade. The mouth sores and digestive issues that plagued me went away as well. But I still struggled with fatigue and brain fog and I knew I hadn't quite gotten to the root of my Hashimoto's. After seeing a chiropractor who specialized in thyroid disorders, I finally got the answers I needed.

Testing revealed an *H. pylori* (helicobacter pylori) infection—one of the gut infections we'll look at more closely in a moment. This infection, like all the infections in the list below, was continuing to trigger an inflammatory response in my body and putting my immune system on overdrive, making it difficult to heal and regain my energy.

It's important to consider the possibility of an underlying infection when your dietary and other lifestyle changes just don't seem to be doing enough to move the needle in terms of getting your energy levels and mood back on track. Certain infections have been found to be more common in those with autoimmune issues specifically, and it's worth finding out if these infections are contributing to your fatigue.

Remember, just because you haven't been diagnosed with a full-blown autoimmune disease, doesn't mean those nagging health issues aren't landing you on the road to one. The general feelings of tiredness, brain fog, depression, anxiety, digestive and skin issues are all signs of imbalance that, left unchecked, have the potential to become more serious problems down the road. Let's look at some of the most common types of infections that may be disrupting your health so that you don't end up with an ugly diagnosis in your future, if you haven't had one already.

Gut Infections

If all disease begins in the gut, then gut infections are of particular concern to our overall health. The following list of toxic infections is by no means exhaustive. However, I wanted to highlight a few of the more common infections that can contribute to low energy and cognitive issues.

H. Pylori

H. pylori is a particularly common and nasty infection that can be difficult to pinpoint since those infected often show no outward symptoms. This bacterium can burrow into the lining of the stomach wall where it suppresses the production of stomach acid, increasing susceptibility to other infections such as parasites.

Not to mention, low stomach acid equates to less efficient digestion, nutrient malabsorption, and leaky gut. Vitamin B12 and iron absorption can be diminished, for example, when stomach acid is suppressed by H. pylori, further perpetuating the cycle of fatigue. So, it's important to find out if this infection is at the root of your own exhaustion and digestive issues. This infection has been linked to stomach ulcers so if you've struggled with ulcers, you may especially want to get tested. H. pylori is diagnosed through either a stool test or a breath test.

SIBO

Small intestinal bacterial overgrowth, or SIBO, is exactly what it sounds like—an overgrowth of bacteria in the small intestine. This can include both harmful bacteria as well as bacteria that would normally be beneficial in the right amounts. Those suffering from SIBO may experience very general digestive issues such as bloating, abdominal discomfort, diarrhea or constipation, gas, and belching.

SIBO has been linked to an increased risk for autoimmune disease as well as contributing to leaky gut, so it's important to get tested for this condition if you're struggling with the digestive issues listed above that don't respond well to changes in diet and lifestyle. Like H. pylori, SIBO can also be diagnosed via breath test, but note that it can be a tricky condition to get rid of, so it's important to retest after the initial treatment to assure that the overgrowth has been eradicated.

Candida Overgrowth

An opportunistic yeast, *Candida* is part of your normal gut flora. When your system is out of balance through eating the wrong foods, Candida seizes its chance to take over, creating symptoms ranging from brain fog and mood swings to digestive issues, sugar cravings and, of course, chronic fungal infections. Just like most of the other toxic infections we've looked at, Candida also contributes to leaky gut, further weakening the immune system and promoting inflammation.

A simple stool test can detect a Candida infection, although blood testing can be used as well. Because sugar feeds Candida, one of the best ways to beat this nasty infection is simply through eating a diet high in quality protein, veggies, and healthy fats and limiting the toxic foods we looked at—especially sugar in all forms, including fruit, honey, and processed sugars.

Because the lauric acid in coconut oil is beneficial in fighting fungal infections, it's also great to incorporate a tablespoon or so a day into your diet when dealing with Candida. A qualified practitioner will also be able to recommend some herbal supplements that can help as well.

Epstein-Barr Virus

Another infection associated with depleted energy levels is the *Epstein-Barr virus* (EBV). If you've ever been diagnosed with *mono* (infectious mononucleosis), it's possible that the Epstein-Barr virus is a contributing factor in your ongoing struggle with fatigue, since the virus that causes mono and the virus that causes EBV are, in fact, one and the same.

Part of the herpes family of viruses, EBV can be present yet dormant in the body so that you could be carrying the virus for years without showing symptoms. It's important to note, however, that just because you haven't had a mono diagnosis, doesn't mean EBV isn't at work. Because of its link to autoimmune diseases, including autoimmune thyroid disease and multiple sclerosis, it's an important factor to consider for anyone struggling with chronic exhaustion and autoimmunity. Your doctor can perform a simple blood test to diagnose this infection.

Dental Infections

Infections in the mouth have been shown to have a link to autoimmune disease and are worth considering when getting to the root of disease caused by chronic inflammation. Cavities, gum disease, and root canals are all potential sources of infectious bacteria which can then be introduced into the body through the bloodstream, inciting an immune response which triggers inflammation.

While any type of dental work poses the risk for infections, root canals are especially susceptible to infection since it's impossible to completely remove all areas of infection from the dead tooth. The likelihood of the root canal harboring infectious agents is extremely high and can allow toxins to seep into the bloodstream and incite inflammation and the autoimmune response.

I experienced this situation first-hand. A lesion I discovered on the roof of my mouth turned out to be an infection from a dying tooth that had tunneled through the bone. My dentist recommended that I have a root canal. I happily agreed, assuming my dentist wouldn't recommend any procedure that would be harmful to my health.

Unfortunately, about a year after the root canal was done, the area again became infected and I chose to have the tooth extracted rather than continue the cycle of "root canal-infection-root canal" that was offered to me. The underlying infection in my mouth was contributing to my autoimmune response and had to go. I've since learned about the dangers of root canals and would caution anyone considering a root canal to do their homework before proceeding.

The Solution to Toxic Infections

The first step in eradicating toxic infections is to get a proper diagnosis in the first place. As already noted, most of these gut infections can be diagnosed through either a stool test or, in the case of H. pylori and SIBO, a breath test.

The problem isn't so much getting the testing done as it is finding a qualified health practitioner who will be willing to do the testing.

I want to take a moment to dive into how to find a qualified practitioner who can help you get to the root of your problem as this may be a deal-breaker in finding a solution to the exhaustion, brain fog, and other health issues you're dealing with. I've heard story after story of patients who have gone from doctor to doctor without finding the solutions they needed before they finally found the one doctor who could put all the pieces into place, get the proper testing done, and finally help the patient heal and regain their life.

In some cases, women have gone to upwards of a dozen or more doctors only to be told there is nothing wrong with them, it's all in their head, or some other type of dismissal that leaves the patient with no hope of feeling better. I want to state emphatically that this type of health care is simply not acceptable. There is **absolutely** an answer to the debilitating fatigue and health issues you feel burdened with. Don't let anyone, including your doctor, tell you everything is fine and your lab tests are normal when you know the fatigue and brain fog are anything but normal.

There are some simple things to look for when searching for a health practitioner to help you find the root cause of your fatigue and I want to share those with you now so you can find the right practitioner quickly and get on your way to amazing health without having to go from one doctor to the next, spending years, not to mention lots of money, without finding a real solution.

Functional Medicine

It's important to realize that there are two types of health care vying for your patient dollars today. The first type of medicine is known as *allopathic* medicine, or what I like to refer to as *conventional medicine*. This is the type of health care most of us grew up with. Conventional medicine refers to the type of health care that treats illness with medical interventions that include pharmaceutical drugs. You have an infection? Here's an antibiotic. Got high blood pressure? We've got statin drugs for that. Whatever your ailment, rest assured, allopathic medicine has a drug for it.

While I have nothing against doctors who practice medicine this way, there are a few inherent problems with treating illness with pharmaceuticals. One of the biggest being that pharmaceutical drugs come with a high price tag. No, I'm not referring to the actual cost you pay in dollars, although we can add that to our list of "problems associated with conventional medicine." The price tag I'm talking about is the one that you pay for with your health.

Most drugs have side effects which are often worse than the disease they are supposed to be treating. I'm not the smartest cookie on the block, but doesn't it seem illogical to take a drug for eczema (an annoying but relatively harmless skin condition) which may cause liver failure, which is *deadly?* Like the food industry, the healthcare industry has become more concerned with grabbing your dollars than with providing for your health. Once again, uninformed consumers are the ones who pay the price.

A Better Way

Fortunately, allopathic medicine isn't your only option when it comes to diagnosing and treating chronic health issues. *Functional medicine* refers to the type of health care where the practitioner looks at your symptoms and illness not as a separate and distinct disease operating apart from your other body systems. Instead, functional medicine looks at the body as a whole.

If you're struggling with depression or thyroid issues, for example, the functional medicine practitioner wants to know what's going on with your gut and with your immune system and how they are all related. Furthermore, unlike conventional medicine, functional medicine concerns itself with getting to the *root* of your illness, rather than just treating the *symptoms* with medications that only mask the true problem.

Thyroid issues are a great example of how conventional medicine and functional medicine differentiate in their treatment of disease. If a woman goes to her (conventional) doctor complaining of fatigue, weight gain, and depression, the doctor will likely check her thyroid levels through a simple blood test. If those tests come back showing that her thyroid is not functioning normally, she'll be given a diagnosis of hypothyroidism and sent happily on her way with a prescription for Synthroid or one of the other thyroid hormone replacement drugs on the market. It's highly likely that the doctor diagnosing and treating the condition won't even mention the patient's dietary habits or gut health—which we've seen are critical issues in treating a thyroid condition.

A functional medicine practitioner, however, takes a more holistic view of the body. Once he recognizes a true thyroid disorder through blood tests, he'll begin to look at the overall health of the patient. He may ask questions about how the patient grew up, health history, as well as her diet and bowel habits—all important clues into the patient's current health status. The functional medicine practitioner will also recognize that treating the patient through dietary interventions, as well as specific supplements including herbals and essential oils, will help to rebalance the gut while also addressing hormonal imbalances.

Finding a Functional Medicine Practitioner

So, how does one go about finding the right health care practitioner? In a sea of doctors, naturopaths, chiropractors, nutritionists, and more, where do you start to look? Heaven knows, going from one practitioner to the next attempting to find the right person can be time consuming and costly. The Institute for Functional Medicine is a great place to start. You'll find a directory of practitioners who are certified in functional medicine on their website at *functionalmedicine.org*.

The Gluten Free Society also has a directory on their website where you can search for a doctor in your area who understands the problems associated with gluten and gut health. You can find their website at *glutenfreesociety.org*. You can find a Certified Gluten Practitioner at www.thedr.com/find-a-certified-gluten-practitioner.

Finally, many chiropractors and naturopaths take a more holistic view of the body and can help you get to the root of fatigue and brain fog by examining which gut issues are playing into your health issues. However, just because someone claims to be a functional medicine practitioner or a holistic practitioner doesn't necessarily mean that they are the right practitioner to help you. I recommend you do your homework, check references, get recommendations, and ask the right questions to find the right health care provider.

Checking out your functional medicine practitioner before you begin working with them is always a good idea. It's important to know, going into the initial consultation, if they are going to be willing to listen to your concerns and help you find the solutions you need. Not all functional medicine practitioners are created equal. I found this out the hard way when I traveled over an hour to see a biological dentist who, as it ends up, practiced dentistry in many ways similar to a conventionally-trained dentist and only worsened the dental infection I was dealing with, rather than treating it properly.

So, what questions should you ask? Start with a few simple questions to get a good idea of who your practitioner is and how they'll work with you. I created a separate guide that includes questions to ask a potential health care professional before deciding if they are a good fit for you to work with. You can download the guide in the bonuses section of this book.

Dentistry

I highly recommend finding a dentist who practices functional medicine as well, since, as we've seen, dental infections and unsafe dental practices, such as placing mercury in the mouth, are often contributors to chronic diseases. When looking for a dentist, I recommend you find a biological dentist, certified by the International Academy of Biological Dentistry and Medicine (IABDM), which you can conveniently locate on their website at www.iabdm.org.

Biological dentistry is concerned with how certain substances in the body affect the overall health of the patient and, in general, is more cautious about the materials used in dental procedures, foregoing toxic compounds (mainly mercury). I've already shared my unfortunate experience with a biological dentist. Use websites, like the IABDM, as a starting point but don't neglect asking the right questions.

Health Coaching

Health coaching is an exciting area of health care that is gaining popularity—and for good reason. A health coach can help bridge the gap between information and implementation. As Dr. Tom O'Bryan shared with me during our interview, the health coach is a critically important component of your health care team that, "walks with you through the mud of transition." Let's face it: it's a lot of work to transition to a healthier lifestyle. It's one thing to know you should eat better—ditch sugar, eat more veggies or buy organic. Ever notice that it's a whole different ball game to put those recommendations into practice? Mmm hmm . . . we're all guilty of this. This is where a health coach can be instrumental in helping you achieve the goals you've set in place for improving your diet and lifestyle habits and getting to the bottom of why those changes can often be so hard to make.

Coaching is a right fit for the person who recognizes that they are responsible for the level of health and success they achieve and who is looking for answers that will truly create positive outcomes in their life rather than just looking for a "quick-fix" solution to their health issues. Health coaches can help their clients see where they are holding themselves back through objective observation and questions. When coaching is combined with the right functional medical interventions, the results can be powerful.

As a health coach, I've seen how powerful it can be for women to have someone in their corner, giving them the tools and information they need to transform their health. The accountability alone is a powerful motivator in helping you reach your goals and when it's combined with the right knowledge, your chances of achieving your health goals increase exponentially.

When you have the right players on your team, you can make progress much more quickly than going it alone. Make sure the health care practitioners you choose share your same philosophy on treating the body and are willing to listen to your concerns and questions. Once you've ruled out and dealt with any underlying infections, you'll be on your way to abundant energy and vibrant health every day!

Conclusion

We've looked at a lot of toxins throughout this book. While I want to remind you that my goal isn't to overwhelm you, I know that can often be our first reaction when we see what we're up against.

I've been there. When I first learned that everything, from what I was eating to what I was putting on my body and, even, the furniture in my home, were potentially making me sick, I felt overwhelmed as well. As I began to study this area of health, it seemed like I learned of something new every week that was toxic and harmful to my health.

My advice is to first let yourself feel those emotions. Give yourself permission to feel the frustration, the exhaustion, the anger. Then, get over it. *Really*. You are bigger than the toxins that are trying to take you out and there is nothing that can truly overwhelm your ability to heal unless you give it permission to.

This book has given you the tools you need to take control of your health and your energy. You know which foods to eat to nourish your DNA, feed your mitochondria and dial down inflammation—and which foods to avoid. You know what to look for when purchasing skin care and cleaning products. You know that your choices in what you think about or how much sleep you get each night are going to affect your energy levels tomorrow—and that it's totally within your power to control those things. You also know how to find the help you need in searching for underlying infections and nutrient deficiencies that may be triggering your exhaustion.

Now it's up to you. I hope you'll take the information presented in this book and use it to truly get to the root of your exhaustion so you can regain the abundant energy and mental clarity that are your birthright. I hope you'll take this opportunity to ditch the quick-fix, pill-popping mentality that we've come to rely on in our face-paced, "have-it-all-now" society.

When you start to live your life with intention, choosing foods because they nourish, making important habits a part of your daily routine, and looking for real answers to your health problems, you'll find yourself opening up to life in a new and exciting way. You'll experience how powerful it is to feel in control of your choices about what you eat—instead of letting food control you. You'll know what it's like to wake up energetic and clear minded—instead of groggy and depressed. You'll experience how good it feels to go through your day feeling great, instead of crashing each afternoon or struggling to fall asleep at night.

Just think of the powerful example you'll be setting for your children as well. I've noticed that, as I've adopted healthier eating habits over the years, my own children have been more open to trying new foods and avoiding certain foods that aren't as healthy. It's an amazing feeling as a mom to watch my children make intentional choices about their health and their bodies. Knowing those habits will serve them through their lifetime is one of the greatest legacies I can give them.

My hope for you is that you won't let the information on these pages just be some nice recommendations you might try someday. Ditching the toxins in the five areas we've discussed totally transformed my health—not just physically, but mentally—and I'm confident it can transform your health as well.

Here's your chance to take control of your health, your mind, and your ability to show up in life as the strong, vibrant woman you long to be. Here's your chance to feel amazing in your body, experience clear skin, clear thinking, and so much more. Be sure to download the <u>bonuses</u> to *Energy Reset* so you can have even more tools at your fingertips to help you reset your hormones and regain your energy.

I've found one of the quickest ways to accelerate my progress in any area is to get around other people who have similar goals and values as myself. I'd love to invite you to join our online community of women who are interested in ditching the toxins, regaining our energy, and living life vibrantly over in the Vibrant Moms Community on Facebook. We'd love to have you, so come join the conversation and let's start ditching the toxins and regaining our energy together!

Selected Bibliography

Wentz, I. *Hashimoto's Thyroiditis: Lifestyle Interventions for Finding and Treating the Root Cause*. Wentz, LLC, 2013.

http://news.nationalgeographic.com/2016/01/160111-microbiome-estimate-count-ratio-human-health-science/

Myers, A. *The Thyroid Connection: Why You Feel Tired, Brain-Fogged, and Overweight— And How to Get Your Life Back*. New York: Little, Brown and Company, 2016.

Christianson, A. *The Adrenal Reset Diet*, New York: Harmony Books, 2014.

Ann Emerg Med. 2007 Jun 21; Does Progesterone Have Neuroprotective Properties? Donald G Stein, David W Wright, Arthur L Kellermann Brain Research Laboratory, Department of Emergency Medicine, School of Medicine (Stein, Wright).

Brogan, K. And K. Loberg. *A Mind of Your Own*. New York: Harper Wave, 2016.

Campbell-McBride, Natasha. *Gut and Psychology Syndrome.* Cambridge: Medinform Publishing, 2004.

Kharrazian, D. Why Do I Still Have Thyroid Symptoms? When My Lab Tests Are Normal. Carlsbad, CA: Elephant Press, 2010.

Axe, J., *Eat Dirt: Why Leaky Gut May Be the Root Cause of Your Health Problems and 5 Surprising Steps to Cure It.* New York: HarperCollins, 2016.

https://draxe.com/cancer-fighting-cla-higher-in-grass-fed-beef/

http://www.safecosmetics.org/wp-content/uploads/2015/02/Not-So-Sexy-report.pdf

Leaf, C. *Switch On Your Brain*, Grand Rapids, MI: Baker Books, 2013.

Cuddy, A. Presence, New York: Little, Brown and Company, 2015.

Kulacz, R., and T. Levy, *The Toxic Tooth*, Henderson, NV: MedFox Publishing, 2014.

https://chriskresser.com/sibo-what-causes-it-and-why-its-so-hard-to-treat/

Acknowledgments

This book wouldn't have been possible without the feedback and support of many people. Thank you to Sarah McLain, RN, for your help and encouragement, as well as to Jaime Boyachek, RN, CTNC, for invaluable insight and feedback on this project.

Thank you to Trina Felber, CEO of Primal Life Organics, as well as Jeffrey Smith and Amy Hart, film makers behind the documentary Secret Ingredients, for their insightful interviews which provided the information for this book. Thank you to Dr. Tom O'Bryan for taking the time to discuss how toxins interfere with the immune system and accelerate the disease process. I would also like to thank Regina Felty for proofreading and editing of the manuscript.

Thank you to my mom, Laura Woodruff, for your unending support and love as I worked on this project. Finally, thank you to my husband and three children who always support me in everything I do.

About the Author

Michelle Brown is a Certified Transformational Nutrition Coach (CTNC) who specializes in helping women with detoxification, hormonal imbalance, and gut and adrenal health. By helping women choose the 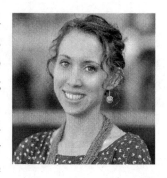 right foods that encourage detoxification and good gut health, as well as teaching them to adopt healthy lifestyle habits that balance the hormones, Michelle shows women how they can reset their energy and rebalance their mental and emotional health. You can find Michelle at www.overcomingauto.com.

Contact Me:
Overcomingauto@gmail.com

If you found *Energy Reset* helpful, would you consider leaving a review on Amazon? Your review will help other women struggling with exhaustion and hormonal imbalance to find the answers they need. Thank you!

65193932R00137

Made in the USA
San Bernardino, CA
28 December 2017